THE ESSENTIAL GUIDE TO CANNABIS EXTRACTS:

A Beginner's Journey into Concentrated Bliss

Contents

1. INTRODUCTION

1.1 Brief Overview of Cannabis

Cannabis, also known as marijuana, is a genus of flowering plants that belong to the Cannabaceae family. The two primary species within the Cannabis genus are Cannabis sativa and Cannabis indica, with hybrid varieties combining characteristics of both. Cannabis has been cultivated for various purposes for thousands of years, and its usage has evolved across cultures.

Key Components:

1. Cannabinoids:

- Cannabis contains over 100 different cannabinoids, with THC (tetrahydrocannabinol) and CBD (cannabidiol) being the most well-known. These compounds interact with the endocannabinoid system in the human body, influencing various physiological processes.

2. Terpenes:

- Terpenes are aromatic compounds found in cannabis that contribute to its distinct flavors and scents. They also play a role in the overall effects of different cannabis strains.

Historical Significance:

- Cannabis has a rich history of use for medicinal, recreational, and industrial purposes. Ancient civilizations in China, India, and the Middle East utilized cannabis for its therapeutic properties.

Cultural and Recreational Use:

- Cannabis has been traditionally used in cultural and religious ceremonies in various parts of the world. In recent times, it has gained popularity for recreational purposes, with users seeking its psychoactive effects.

Medicinal Applications:

- Cannabis has been studied for its potential medicinal benefits. It is used to alleviate symptoms associated with conditions such as chronic pain, nausea, and certain neurological disorders. The medicinal use of cannabis is a topic of ongoing research and evolving legal frameworks.

Legislation and Regulation:

- The legal status of cannabis varies globally. Some regions have legalized it for medical and/or recreational use, while others maintain strict regulations or prohibition. Changes in legislation and public perception have influenced the evolving landscape of cannabis use.

Cultivation and Varieties:

- Cannabis plants can be cultivated both indoors and outdoors. Different strains exhibit varying ratios of cannabinoids and terpenes, leading to distinct effects. Sativa strains are often associated with uplifting effects, while indica strains may be more relaxing.

Challenges and Opportunities:

- The legalization and regulation of cannabis pose challenges and opportunities for governments, industries, and individuals. The plant's diverse uses, coupled with ongoing research, contribute to a dynamic and evolving understanding of cannabis and its potential impact on society.

1.2 Evolution of Cannabis Consumption

Cannabis consumption has a long and multifaceted history, shaped by cultural, social, and legal factors. The ways in which cannabis is used have evolved significantly over time, reflecting changes in societal attitudes, technological advancements, and scientific understanding. Here is a brief overview of the evolution of cannabis consumption:

Ancient and Traditional Use:

- Early Medicinal and Ritualistic Use: Cannabis has been used for medicinal and ritualistic purposes for thousands of years. Ancient civilizations in China,

India, and the Middle East incorporated cannabis into traditional medicine and religious ceremonies.

Pre-20th Century:

- Global Medicinal Use: Cannabis continued to be utilized for its medicinal properties, with tinctures and extracts commonly prescribed for a range of ailments in the 19th century.
- Introduction to the West: Cannabis was introduced to Western medicine in the 19th century, leading to its inclusion in various pharmaceutical products.

20th Century:

- Prohibition Era: The early 20th century saw the rise of cannabis prohibition in many parts of the world, influenced by moral, racial, and political factors. This led to the criminalization of cannabis use, cultivation, and distribution.

- Counterculture Movement: In the mid-20th century, cannabis became associated with the counterculture movement. The 1960s and 1970s saw increased recreational use, often in the form of smoking.

Late 20th Century:

- Medical Cannabis Movement: The latter half of the 20th century saw a resurgence of interest in the medicinal properties of cannabis. Patients and advocates began pushing for the legalization of medical cannabis to alleviate symptoms associated with various medical conditions.

21st Century:

- Legalization and Regulation: The 21st century witnessed a shift in attitudes towards cannabis. Some regions began legalizing cannabis for medical and recreational use, acknowledging its potential benefits and generating new economic opportunities.
- Diversification of Products: Advancements in extraction technologies led to the creation of a wide range of cannabis products beyond traditional smoking, including edibles, tinctures, topicals, and concentrates.
- Cannabis in Wellness: Cannabis has entered the wellness industry, with CBD products gaining popularity for their perceived health benefits. This has contributed to a more mainstream acceptance of certain cannabis-derived compounds.

Ongoing Trends:

- Research and Education: Ongoing scientific research is contributing to a better understanding of cannabinoids, terpenes, and their effects on the human body. Education efforts aim to inform consumers about responsible and informed cannabis use.

- Global Perspectives: Cannabis legalization and regulation continue to evolve globally, with varying approaches and policies in different regions.
- The evolution of cannabis consumption reflects a complex interplay of cultural, social, and scientific factors, and its trajectory is likely to continue evolving in response to changing societal norms and advancements in research and technology.

1.3 Purpose of Cannabis Extracts

Cannabis extracts serve a variety of purposes, ranging from medicinal applications to recreational use. The extraction process isolates and concentrates the beneficial compounds from the cannabis plant, offering users more precise and potent options compared to traditional consumption methods. Here are some key purposes of cannabis extracts:

1. Medicinal Benefits:

- Targeted Treatment: Cannabis extracts allow for the isolation of specific cannabinoids, such as CBD (cannabidiol) or THC (tetrahydrocannabinol), which can be used to address specific medical conditions, including chronic pain, inflammation, seizures, and anxiety.
- Precise Dosage: Extracts enable patients to consume precise doses of cannabinoids, facilitating better control over their treatment regimens.

2. Diverse Consumption Methods:

- Versatility: Cannabis extracts can be incorporated into various products, including tinctures, edibles, topicals, and capsules. This versatility provides consumers with multiple consumption options based on their preferences and needs.

3. Reduced Inhalation Risks:

- Avoidance of Smoking: Extracts offer an alternative to smoking, reducing the potential risks associated with inhaling combusted plant material. Vaporizing and edibles, for example, provide smoke-free consumption methods.

4. Convenience and Portability:

- Ease of Use: Extracts are often more concentrated than raw cannabis flower, allowing for smaller, more manageable doses. This can be particularly convenient for users seeking a discreet and portable method of consumption.

5. Enhanced Flavor and Aroma:

- Terpene Preservation: Extraction methods can preserve the plant's terpenes, which contribute to its distinctive flavors and aromas. This allows consumers to experience a more nuanced and flavorful profile compared to some traditional consumption methods.

6. Economical and Efficient:

-   Higher Potency: Cannabis extracts can be significantly more potent than raw cannabis flower, meaning users may need less material to achieve the desired effects. This efficiency can make extracts a cost-effective option for both medicinal and recreational users.

7. Recreational Use:

-   Diverse Products: Cannabis extracts offer recreational users a wide array of products, including concentrates like shatter, wax, and oils, which can be used in various ways, such as dabbing or vaping.

8. Customization for Wellness:

-   Tailored Experiences: Cannabis extracts allow users to customize their experiences by selecting products with specific cannabinoid and terpene profiles. This customization is especially relevant for those seeking particular effects, such as relaxation or focus.

9. Research and Development:

- Scientific Exploration: Extracts provide researchers with standardized and controlled substances for scientific studies, contributing to a deeper understanding of the therapeutic potential of cannabinoids and other cannabis compounds.

10. Compliance with Regulations:

- Standardized Products: In regions where cannabis is regulated, extracts provide a standardized way to deliver consistent doses, ensuring compliance with legal requirements and quality standards.

2. UNDERSTANDING CANNABIS

2.1 Cannabis Plant Anatomy

Understanding the anatomy of the cannabis plant is crucial for both cultivators and consumers. Here's an overview of the basic components of the cannabis plant:

1. Roots:

- Function: Anchors the plant in the soil and absorbs water and nutrients.
- Characteristics: The root system is extensive, with a central taproot and numerous lateral roots.

2. Stem:

- Function: Provides structural support and transports water, nutrients, and sugars.
- Characteristics: The main stem has nodes where branches, leaves, and buds emerge.

3. Nodes:

- Function: Sites on the stem where branches, leaves, and buds grow.
- Characteristics: Nodes are critical for the plant's growth and flowering, with alternating patterns along the stem.

4. Leaves:

- Function: Primary sites for photosynthesis, producing sugars and oxygen.
- Characteristics: Cannabis leaves are typically palmate with serrated edges, and the number of leaflets varies between different cannabis species and strains.

5. Fan Leaves:

- Function: Larger leaves that provide a broad surface area for photosynthesis.
- Characteristics: Fan leaves are crucial for capturing sunlight and converting it into energy.

6. Trichomes:

- Function: Tiny, hair-like structures that produce cannabinoids and terpenes.
- Characteristics: Trichomes give the plant a "frosted" appearance and are especially concentrated on the flowers (buds).

7. Buds (Flowers):

- Function: The reproductive structures where cannabinoids and terpenes are most concentrated.
- Characteristics: Buds vary in size, density, and color, depending on the strain. They are harvested for medicinal and recreational use.

8. Calyx:

- Function: Protective layer around the reproductive organs within the bud.
- Characteristics: Calyxes are often resinous and play a role in determining the plant's overall potency.

9. Pistils:

- Function: Female reproductive organs that capture pollen for fertilization.
- Characteristics: Pistils are hair-like structures emerging from the calyxes and change color as the plant matures.

10. Stigma:

- Function: Part of the female reproductive system, designed to capture pollen.
- Characteristics: Stigmas are often visible as the brightly colored hairs on female flowers.

11. Cola:

- Function: A cluster of buds on the same stem.
- Characteristics: The main cola is typically the largest and most mature cluster, while smaller colas develop on side branches.

12. Sugar Leaves:

- Function: Surround buds and may contain trichomes.
- Characteristics: Smaller leaves that are often covered in resin, contributing to the overall potency.

2.2 Types of Cannabis: Sativa, Indica, and Hybrid

Cannabis plants are commonly categorized into three main types: Sativa, Indica, and Hybrid. These classifications are based on the plant's morphology, growth characteristics, and reported effects. It's important to note that these distinctions are not always clear-cut, as many modern strains are hybrids with characteristics of both Sativa and Indica. Here's an overview of each type:

1. Sativa:

- Appearance:
- Taller and slimmer plants with long, narrow leaves.
- Sparse foliage, allowing light to penetrate to lower branches.
- Growth Characteristics:
- Longer flowering time (10-16 weeks).
- Thrives in warmer climates with a longer growing season.
- Effects:
- Typically associated with uplifting and energizing effects.

- Often used during the day for increased creativity, focus, and sociability.
- Common Uses:
- Daytime use, socializing, creative activities, and managing mood disorders.

2. Indica:

- Appearance:
- Shorter, bushier plants with wider leaves.
- Dense foliage, creating a more compact appearance.
- Growth Characteristics:
- Shorter flowering time (8-12 weeks).
- Well-suited for indoor cultivation and shorter growing seasons.
- Effects:
- Generally associated with relaxing and sedative effects.
- Often used in the evening or before bedtime for relaxation and sleep aid.
- Common Uses:
- Nighttime use, stress relief, relaxation, and managing insomnia or pain.

3. Hybrid:

- Genetic Combination:
- Hybrids are a mix of Sativa and Indica genetics.
- The ratio of Sativa to Indica can vary, and effects depend on the specific hybrid strain.

- Appearance:
- Traits may lean toward either Sativa or Indica, depending on the genetic dominance.
- Growth Characteristics:
- Flowering time and growth patterns vary based on the specific hybrid strain.
- Effects:
- Hybrid effects can be balanced or may lean more toward one type, depending on the strain.
- Hybrids offer a wide range of effects, catering to diverse consumer preferences.
- Common Uses:
- Depending on the dominant traits, hybrids can be suitable for various purposes, from relaxation to creative stimulation.

It's essential to recognize that the Sativa-Indica classification system has limitations, and individual experiences may vary. Additionally, the chemical profile, including the concentrations of cannabinoids and terpenes, plays a significant role in the effects of a particular strain. As the cannabis industry evolves, more emphasis is placed on analyzing these chemical profiles to provide a more accurate representation of a strain's potential effects.

2.3 Cannabinoids and Their Effects

Cannabinoids are chemical compounds found in the cannabis plant that interact with the endocannabinoid system (ECS) in the human body. The ECS plays a crucial role in regulating various physiological processes, including mood, appetite, sleep, and immune function. The two main types of cannabinoids are endocannabinoids (produced naturally in the body) and phytocannabinoids (found in cannabis). Here are some key cannabinoids found in cannabis and their general effects:

1. Tetrahydrocannabinol (THC):

- Effect: Psychoactive, produces the "high" associated with cannabis.
- Medical Uses: Pain relief, appetite stimulation, nausea reduction, muscle spasm reduction.
- Other Effects: Euphoria, relaxation, altered perception of time and space.

2. Cannabidiol (CBD):

- Effect: Non-psychoactive, does not produce a "high."
- Medical Uses: Anti-inflammatory, analgesic (pain relief), anxiolytic (anxiety reduction), antipsychotic, anti-seizure.
- Other Effects: Relaxation, improved mood, potential neuroprotective properties.

3. Cannabinol (CBN):

- Effect: Mildly psychoactive, often associated with sedation.

- Medical Uses: Sleep aid, anti-inflammatory, potential appetite stimulation.
- Other Effects: Relaxation, potential anti-bacterial properties.

4. Cannabigerol (CBG):

- Effect: Non-psychoactive, precursor to other cannabinoids.
- Medical Uses: Anti-inflammatory, potential neuroprotective effects, appetite stimulation.
- Other Effects: Relaxation.

5. Cannabichromene (CBC):

- Effect: Non-psychoactive.
- Medical Uses: Anti-inflammatory, potential pain relief, anti-fungal.
- Other Effects: Potential antidepressant properties.

6. Tetrahydrocannabivarin (THCV):

- Effect: Psychoactive in high doses, may have a stimulating effect.
- Medical Uses: Potential appetite suppression, anti-convulsant, potential anti-inflammatory.
- Other Effects: May have energizing effects.

7. Cannabidivarin (CBDV):

- Effect: Non-psychoactive.
- Medical Uses: Anti-epileptic, potential anti-nausea effects.
- Other Effects: Research is ongoing to explore additional therapeutic applications.

8. Delta-8-THC:

- Effect: Psychoactive but less potent than Delta-9-THC.
- Medical Uses: Similar to Delta-9-THC, including pain relief and appetite stimulation.
- Other Effects: Euphoria, relaxation.

The effects of cannabinoids can vary based on factors such as the specific cannabinoid, its concentration in the product, the presence of other cannabinoids and terpenes, and individual differences in metabolism and sensitivity. Understanding the diverse effects of cannabinoids is crucial for both medical and recreational cannabis users to make informed choices based on their preferences and desired outcomes.

3. WHAT ARE CANNABIS EXTRACTS?

3.1 Definition and Basics

Definition:

Cannabis, also known as marijuana, is a genus of flowering plants in the Cannabaceae family. The primary species are Cannabis sativa, Cannabis indica, and Cannabis ruderalis. The plant has been used for various purposes for thousands of years, including medicinal, recreational, industrial, and spiritual uses.

Key Components:

1. Cannabinoids:

   - Cannabis produces over 100 different cannabinoids, with THC (tetrahydrocannabinol) and CBD (cannabidiol) being the most well-known. These compounds interact with the endocannabinoid system in the human body, influencing various physiological processes.

2. Terpenes:

   - Terpenes are aromatic compounds found in cannabis that contribute to its distinctive flavors and scents. They also play a role in the overall effects of different cannabis strains.

Cannabis Plant Basics:

1. Cultivation:

- Cannabis can be cultivated both indoors and outdoors, with specific environmental conditions influencing plant growth. The cultivation process includes germination, vegetative growth, flowering, and harvesting.

2. Male and Female Plants:

- Cannabis plants are typically dioecious, meaning they have separate male and female plants. Female plants produce flowers (buds), which are sought after for their higher cannabinoid content.

3. Flowers (Buds):

- The flowers or buds of the female cannabis plant contain the highest concentrations of cannabinoids, including THC and CBD. These compounds are responsible for the plant's psychoactive and medicinal effects.

4. Harvesting:

- The timing of harvesting is crucial to the potency and effects of the cannabis. Harvesting too early or too late can impact the cannabinoid and terpene profiles of the plant.

Modes of Consumption:

1. Smoking:

- Inhaling the smoke from burning cannabis flowers is one of the most traditional and common methods of consumption.

2. Vaporizing:

- Vaporizers heat cannabis to a temperature that releases cannabinoids and terpenes without combustion, reducing the harmful effects of smoking.

3. Edibles:

- Cannabis-infused products, such as brownies or gummies, provide an alternative to smoking for those who prefer not to inhale.

4. Topicals:

- Creams, balms, and lotions infused with cannabinoids for localized relief without the psychoactive effects.

5. Tinctures:

-   Liquid extracts of cannabis, often placed under the tongue for faster absorption.

6. Dabbing:

-   Inhaling vaporized cannabis concentrates, such as wax or shatter, using a specialized rig.

Legal Considerations:

-   The legality of cannabis varies globally and regionally. Some places have legalized cannabis for medical and/or recreational use, while others maintain strict regulations or prohibition.

3.2 Different Forms of Cannabis Extracts

Cannabis extracts come in various forms, each offering unique characteristics and methods of consumption. These extracts concentrate the cannabinoids, terpenes, and other beneficial compounds found in the cannabis plant. Here are some common forms of cannabis extracts:

1. Hashish:

-   Description: Hashish, or hash, is one of the oldest forms of cannabis concentrate. It is made by compressing trichomes (resin glands) from the cannabis plant into a solid, often brown or black, substance.

- Consumption: Hashish is traditionally smoked, either in a pipe, a joint, or mixed with tobacco.

2. Kief:

- Description: Kief consists of the trichome glands that have been separated from the cannabis plant. It has a powdery, crystalline appearance and is rich in cannabinoids and terpenes.
- Consumption: Often added to joints, bowls, or vaporized for an extra potent experience.

3. Tinctures:

- Description: Tinctures are liquid extracts of cannabis that are typically alcohol-based. They allow for precise dosing and are discreet.
- Consumption: Tinctures are usually taken sublingually (under the tongue) for faster absorption, but they can also be added to food or beverages.

4. Cannabis Oil:

- Description: Cannabis oil is an extraction of cannabinoids and terpenes using various solvents. It can be high in THC, CBD, or a combination of both.

- Consumption: Cannabis oil can be ingested, added to edibles, or used in cooking. It is also used in vaporizer pens.

5. Shatter:

- Description: Shatter is a type of cannabis concentrate that is translucent and glass-like in appearance. It is made through a process that involves extracting cannabinoids with a solvent.
- Consumption: Shatter is commonly vaporized or "dabbed" using a specialized rig.

6. Wax:

- Description: Wax, or budder, is a softer and more malleable form of cannabis concentrate. It has a creamy, wax-like texture and is rich in cannabinoids.
- Consumption: Like shatter, wax is often vaporized or dabbed.

7. Live Resin:

- Description: Live resin is made from freshly harvested cannabis plants that are frozen immediately after cutting. This process preserves a higher concentration of terpenes.

- Consumption: Live resin is commonly vaporized or dabbed for an intense flavor experience.

8. CO2 Oil:

- Description: CO2 oil is produced using carbon dioxide as a solvent. This method allows for the extraction of cannabinoids and terpenes without the need for potentially harmful solvents.
- Consumption: CO2 oil is versatile and can be used in vaporizers, edibles, or topicals.

9. Distillate:

- Description: Distillate is a purified form of cannabis extract that is often refined to contain a specific cannabinoid, such as THC or CBD, in high concentrations.
- Consumption: Distillate is commonly used in vape cartridges, edibles, or applied directly under the tongue.

10. Rosin:

- Description: Rosin is a solventless concentrate produced by applying heat and pressure to cannabis flowers or hash. It is a sticky, sap-like substance.
- Consumption: Rosin can be dabbed, vaporized, or added to joints or bowls.

3.3 Popular Extraction Methods

Cannabis extraction is a process that isolates and concentrates the desirable compounds, including cannabinoids and terpenes, from the plant material. Various extraction methods are employed in the cannabis industry, each with its advantages and considerations. Here are some popular cannabis extraction methods:

1. Solvent-Based Extraction:

- Description: Solvents, such as butane, ethanol, or CO_2, are used to dissolve and extract cannabinoids and terpenes from the plant material. The solvent is then evaporated, leaving behind the concentrated extract.
- Advantages: Can produce high yields and diverse extracts.
- Considerations: Ensuring complete solvent removal is crucial for safety. CO_2 extraction is considered safer due to the lack of residual solvents.

2. CO2 Extraction:

- Description: Carbon dioxide is used as a solvent to extract cannabinoids and terpenes. This method can be tuned to extract specific compounds by adjusting temperature and pressure.
- Advantages: No residual solvents, allows for precise control over the extraction process, and preserves terpene profiles well.

- Considerations: Equipment costs can be higher compared to other methods.

3. Hydrocarbon Extraction (Butane, Propane):

- Description: Butane or propane is used as a solvent to extract cannabinoids and terpenes. The solvent is then purged through evaporation.
- Advantages: Efficient extraction process, can produce high-quality concentrates.
- Considerations: Safety precautions are crucial due to the flammable nature of hydrocarbons. Proper purging is necessary to remove residual solvents.

4. Ethanol Extraction:

- Description: Ethanol is used as a solvent to extract cannabinoids and terpenes. The extract is then evaporated, leaving behind the concentrated product.
- Advantages: Generally regarded as safe, cost-effective, and can produce full-spectrum extracts.
- Considerations: Careful control of temperature is required to prevent the extraction of undesirable compounds.

5. Rosin Pressing:

- Description: This solventless method involves applying heat and pressure to cannabis flowers or hash to extract cannabinoids and terpenes.

- Advantages: No use of solvents, simple process that can be done at home, retains terpenes well.
- Considerations: Yields may be lower compared to solvent-based methods.

6. Isopropyl Alcohol (IPA) Extraction:

- Description: Isopropyl alcohol is used as a solvent to extract cannabinoids and terpenes, similar to ethanol extraction.
- Advantages: Cost-effective and efficient.
- Considerations: Purity of the final product depends on the quality of the starting material and the extraction process.

7. Pressurized Hot Water Extraction:

- Description: Hot water under pressure is used to extract cannabinoids and terpenes.
- Advantages: Considered a "green" method as it doesn't use harmful solvents.
- Considerations: May require additional steps to refine the extract.

8. Ultrasonic Extraction:

- Description: Ultrasonic waves are used to break down cell walls and extract cannabinoids and terpenes.
- Advantages: Rapid extraction, minimal heat, and can preserve volatile compounds.
- Considerations: Equipment costs can be relatively high.

The choice of extraction method depends on various factors, including the desired end product, safety considerations, and the specific characteristics of the cannabis strain being processed. Each method has its strengths and limitations, and ongoing research and technological advancements continue to refine these extraction processes.

4. TYPES OF CANNABIS EXTRACTS

4.1 Hashish

Hashish, commonly referred to as "hash," is a cannabis concentrate made from the resin glands (trichomes) of the cannabis plant. These resin glands contain high concentrations of cannabinoids, including THC (tetrahydrocannabinol) and other psychoactive compounds.

Production:

1. Collection: Hash is produced by collecting the resin glands from the cannabis plant. This can involve methods such as dry sifting or using ice water to separate trichomes from the plant material.

2. Compression: Once collected, the resin glands are typically pressed into a solid, block-like form. The compression process transforms the loose trichomes into a dense and cohesive mass.

Appearance:

Hashish can take various forms, and its appearance depends on factors such as the extraction method, the strain of cannabis used, and the region of production. Common forms include:

- Traditional Hand-Pressed Hash: This type is often dark brown or black in color and has a firm texture. It is manually pressed into blocks or bricks.

- Bubble Hash: Created using ice water and mesh screens, bubble hash has a lighter color and a more granular texture compared to traditional hash.

- Hash Oil: In some regions, hashish is further processed into hash oil, a concentrated liquid form that is often used in vaporizers or dabbing.

Consumption:

Hashish is typically consumed by smoking. It can be crumbled and added to joints or pipes, mixed with tobacco, or vaporized. In regions where it is legal, hash oil may be used in vaporizer pens or for dabbing.

Effects:

The effects of hashish are similar to those of cannabis but can be more potent due to the higher concentrations of cannabinoids. Users often experience a euphoric and relaxed state, altered perception of time, and an increased sensitivity to sensory stimuli.

Legality:

The legal status of hashish varies globally and is often aligned with the legal status of cannabis. In some regions, hashish may be legally available for medicinal or recreational use, while in others, it remains prohibited.

Considerations:

1. Quality: The quality of hashish depends on factors such as the strain of cannabis, the extraction method, and the level of impurities. High-quality hash is often valued for its potency and flavor profile.

2. Cultural Significance: Hashish has a long history of cultural and religious significance in various regions, particularly in the Middle East and South Asia. It has been used in traditional rituals and ceremonies for centuries.

It's important to note that, like cannabis, the use of hashish should be approached responsibly and in accordance with local laws and regulations. Additionally, the potential health risks associated with smoking any substance should be considered.

4.2 Kief

Kief is a concentrated form of cannabis, specifically the resinous trichomes (tiny, hair-like structures) that contain cannabinoids, terpenes, and other compounds. It is often referred to as the "crystals" or "crystal resin" found on the surface of cannabis flowers.

Production:

Kief is naturally present on mature cannabis flowers, but it can be collected and separated from the plant material through various methods:

1. Dry Sifting: Cannabis flowers are mechanically agitated, causing the trichomes to fall off. The separated kief is then collected through screens or filters.

2. Grinder Collection: Many cannabis enthusiasts use grinders equipped with a fine mesh screen to catch kief as they break down the flowers. Over time, a significant amount of kief accumulates in the grinder's bottom chamber.

3. Ice Water Extraction: This method involves using ice water to freeze and separate trichomes from the plant material. The extracted kief is then collected and dried.

Appearance:

Kief has a distinctive appearance, resembling a fine, powdery substance with a crystalline texture. It ranges in color from light tan to green, depending on factors such as the cannabis strain and the collection method.

Potency:

Kief is potent because it contains a high concentration of cannabinoids, particularly THC. Since it consists primarily of trichomes, which house cannabinoids and terpenes, it offers a concentrated form of the plant's psychoactive and therapeutic compounds.

Consumption:

Kief can be consumed in various ways:

1. Sprinkled on Cannabis Flower: Many users sprinkle kief on top of cannabis buds before rolling them into a joint or packing them into a pipe or bowl. This enhances the potency of the overall smoking experience.
2. Pressing into Hash: Kief can be pressed into more solid forms, resembling traditional hashish, for alternative consumption methods.
3. Vaporization: Some vaporizers are designed to accommodate concentrates, including kief.

Vaporizing kief provides a cleaner inhalation method compared to smoking.

4. Edibles: Kief can be incorporated into edible recipes, adding potency to a wide range of infused dishes.

Effects:

The effects of consuming kief are similar to those of cannabis, but users may experience more pronounced effects due to the concentrated levels of cannabinoids. Users often report enhanced euphoria, relaxation, and an altered perception of time and space.

Considerations:

1. Storage: Kief should be stored in a cool, dark place to preserve its potency and prevent degradation.

2. Quality: The quality of kief depends on the quality of the cannabis from which it is derived. High-quality, well-preserved cannabis flowers will yield more potent kief.

3. Responsibility: Like any cannabis product, using kief should be done responsibly, keeping in mind individual tolerance levels and the potential for

increased potency compared to regular cannabis flower.

42

Kief is a versatile and potent cannabis concentrate that offers users the opportunity to enhance their cannabis experience in various ways.

4.3 Tinctures

A cannabis tincture is a liquid extract of cannabinoids, primarily THC (tetrahydrocannabinol) and CBD (cannabidiol), obtained through the use of alcohol or glycerin as a solvent. Tinctures are a discreet and convenient way to consume cannabinoids and are known for their versatility and ease of use.

Production:

The production of cannabis tinctures involves extracting cannabinoids from cannabis plant material using alcohol or glycerin. The process typically includes the following steps:

1. Decarboxylation: If the tincture is intended to be psychoactive, the cannabis material is often decarboxylated (heated) to convert THCA (non-psychoactive) into THC (psychoactive).

2. Extraction: The cannabis material is soaked in alcohol or glycerin to extract cannabinoids and other beneficial compounds.

3. Straining: After a designated soaking period, the plant material is strained or filtered to remove solids.

4. Storage: The liquid extract is then stored in a dark, airtight container to preserve its potency.

Consumption:

Cannabis tinctures offer versatile consumption options:

1. Sublingual Administration: Tinctures can be placed under the tongue for sublingual absorption. This method allows for fast absorption directly into the bloodstream, resulting in relatively quick onset of effects.

2. Addition to Food or Beverages: Tinctures can be easily added to food or beverages, providing a discreet way to consume cannabinoids without the need for smoking or vaporization.

3. Topical Application: While not typically consumed orally, cannabis tinctures can be diluted and applied topically for localized relief from conditions such as pain or inflammation.

Advantages of Tinctures:

1. Precise Dosage: Tinctures allow for precise dosing, as the user can control the amount of liquid consumed.

2. Discreet Consumption: Tinctures are discreet and easy to carry, making them a convenient option for users who want to consume cannabis without drawing attention.

3. Onset Time: Sublingual administration provides a faster onset time compared to edibles, allowing users to feel the effects more quickly.

4. Versatility: Tinctures are versatile and can be incorporated into various consumption methods, providing flexibility for users.

Effects:

The effects of cannabis tinctures vary depending on the cannabinoid profile and the individual's tolerance. Generally, users may experience relaxation, euphoria, and relief from symptoms such as pain or anxiety.

Considerations:

1. Dosage: It's essential to start with a low dosage and gradually increase if needed, as the effects can be potent.

2. Storage: Tinctures should be stored in a cool, dark place to prevent degradation of cannabinoids.

3. Alcohol vs. Glycerin: Some users prefer glycerin-based tinctures, especially if they want to avoid alcohol. However, alcohol-based tinctures are more common and often have a longer shelf life.

4. Strain Selection: The strain of cannabis used in the tincture can influence the overall effects, with different strains offering varying cannabinoid and terpene profiles.

Cannabis tinctures provide a discreet and flexible option for individuals seeking the therapeutic benefits of cannabinoids. As with any cannabis product, it's important to be aware of local regulations and use tinctures responsibly.

4.4 Cannabis Oil

Cannabis oil refers to any concentrated extract of the cannabis plant that is rich in cannabinoids, terpenes, and other beneficial compounds. The term is broad and can encompass various types of oils, including those with high THC (tetrahydrocannabinol), high CBD (cannabidiol), or a balanced ratio of cannabinoids.

Production:

Cannabis oil is produced through an extraction process that separates cannabinoids and other compounds from the cannabis plant. Common extraction methods include:

1. Solvent-Based Extraction: Cannabis is soaked in a solvent (such as ethanol, butane, or CO2) to extract cannabinoids. The solvent is then evaporated, leaving behind the concentrated oil.

2. CO2 Extraction: Carbon dioxide is used as a solvent to extract cannabinoids, terpenes, and other compounds. This method is known for its precision and the ability to produce high-quality oils.

3. Olive Oil Extraction: This is a non-solvent method where cannabis is infused with olive oil, and the cannabinoids are extracted into the oil. While this method

is less concentrated than others, it is simpler and can be done at home.

Types of Cannabis Oil:

1. Full-Spectrum Cannabis Oil:

- Contains a broad spectrum of cannabinoids, terpenes, and other beneficial compounds found in the cannabis plant.

- May include THC, CBD, and other cannabinoids in varying proportions.

- Users may experience the entourage effect, where the combined compounds enhance each other's effects.

2. CBD Oil:

- Primarily contains cannabidiol (CBD) with minimal or no THC.

- Non-psychoactive and often used for its potential therapeutic benefits without the "high" associated with THC.

- Available in various ratios of CBD to THC.

3. THC Oil:

- Contains a higher concentration of tetrahydrocannabinol (THC), the psychoactive compound in cannabis.

- Often used for recreational purposes or for medicinal purposes where THC's psychoactive effects are desired.

4. Distillate:

- A refined form of cannabis oil that undergoes additional processing to isolate specific cannabinoids.

- Distillates can be high in THC, CBD, or other cannabinoids, depending on the desired end product.

5. Rick Simpson Oil (RSO):

- Named after Rick Simpson, who popularized its use, RSO is a high-THC oil known for its potential medicinal benefits.

- Often produced using a solvent-based extraction method.

Consumption:

1. Oral Ingestion: Cannabis oil can be taken orally, either directly or by adding it to food or beverages. Effects may take longer to onset compared to smoking or vaporization.

2. Sublingual Administration: Placing drops of oil under the tongue allows for faster absorption into the bloodstream, providing a quicker onset of effects.

3. Topical Application: Some cannabis oils are formulated for topical use, providing localized relief for conditions like pain or inflammation.

4. Vaporization: Cannabis oil can be vaporized using a vaporizer pen or a vaporization device, offering a smoke-free method of consumption.

Effects:

The effects of cannabis oil depend on the specific cannabinoid profile, dosage, and individual factors. THC-dominant oils may produce psychoactive effects, while CBD-dominant oils are generally non-psychoactive and may offer calming or anti-inflammatory effects.

Considerations:

1. Dosage: Careful consideration of dosage is crucial to avoid overconsumption, especially with THC-dominant oils.

2. Regulatory Compliance: Users should be aware of local regulations regarding the legal status of cannabis and cannabis products.

3. Source and Quality: Choose reputable sources for cannabis oil to ensure product quality and safety.

4. Personal Tolerance: Individual tolerance to cannabinoids varies, and users should start with a low dose and adjust as needed.

Cannabis oil is a versatile and potent form of cannabis that offers various options for both recreational and medicinal users. As with any cannabis product, responsible use and adherence to local regulations are important considerations.

4.5 Shatter, Wax, and Other Concentrates

Cannabis concentrates are highly potent extracts that contain elevated levels of cannabinoids, such as THC and CBD, as well as terpenes and other compounds. They come in various forms, each with its unique characteristics and methods of consumption. Here are some popular cannabis concentrates:

1. Shatter:

- Description: Shatter is a translucent, glass-like concentrate that shatters into pieces when broken. Its name comes from its brittle texture.
- Production: Made using a solvent-based extraction method, typically using butane or CO2.
- Consumption: Often vaporized or "dabbed" using a specialized rig. Can also be melted and added to joints or bowls.

2. Wax:

- Description: Wax, or budder, has a softer, more malleable consistency compared to shatter. It has a creamy or waxy texture.
- Production: Similar to shatter, but the extraction process and post-processing steps can result in a waxier consistency.
- Consumption: Vaporized or dabbed. Some users also crumble wax onto joints or bowls.

3. Live Resin:

- Description: Live resin is made from fresh, flash-frozen cannabis plants. This process preserves a higher concentration of terpenes, resulting in a more flavorful extract.
- Production: Flash-freezing the plant material before extraction.
- Consumption: Vaporized or dabbed for a rich and flavorful experience.

4. Crumble:

- Description: Crumble has a dry and crumbly texture, making it easy to handle. It is similar to wax but with a more granular consistency.
- Production: Typically made using a similar extraction process as wax, but with different post-processing techniques.
- Consumption: Vaporized or dabbed. Crumble can also be added to joints or bowls.

5. Rosin:

- Description: Rosin is a solventless concentrate produced by applying heat and pressure to cannabis flowers or hash. It has a sticky, sap-like consistency.
- Production: No solvents are used; instead, heat and pressure are applied to the cannabis material.

- Consumption: Vaporized or dabbed. Rosin can also be added to joints or bowls.

6. Hash:

- Description: Hashish, or hash, is a traditional cannabis concentrate made by compressing trichomes into a solid, often dark-colored substance.
- Production: Typically made through dry sifting or ice water extraction to separate trichomes from the plant material.
- Consumption: Traditionally smoked in pipes or joints. Can also be vaporized or added to joints.

7. Distillate:

- Description: Distillate is a highly refined form of cannabis extract that often appears as a clear or light-colored liquid. It is purified to contain specific cannabinoids.
- Production: Typically involves distillation to isolate and concentrate cannabinoids.
- Consumption: Used in vape cartridges, edibles, or applied directly under the tongue.

8. Sauce:

- Description: Cannabis sauce contains both a liquid portion (terpenes and cannabinoids) and crystalline structures. The result is a flavorful and potent concentrate.

- Production: Produced through a combination of solvent-based extraction and post-processing techniques.
- Consumption: Vaporized or dabbed for a full-spectrum experience.

9. Diamonds:

- Description: Diamond concentrates consist of isolated THC or CBD crystals that resemble diamonds. These crystals are often found in a sauce.
- Production: The process involves crystallization, separating cannabinoids into crystal formations.
- Consumption: Vaporized or dabbed. The combination of diamonds and sauce provides a potent and flavorful experience.

Considerations:

- Potency: Concentrates are highly potent, and users should be mindful of dosage to avoid overconsumption.
- Methods of Consumption: Concentrates are commonly vaporized or dabbed, but some can also be added to joints, bowls, or used in edibles.
- Quality: The quality of concentrates can vary, and users should choose reputable sources to ensure product safety and efficacy.

It's crucial to be informed about the specific type of concentrate, its production methods, and its effects before trying a new product. Additionally, responsible use and adherence to local regulations are essential considerations when consuming cannabis concentrates.

5. CANNABINOIDS AND TERPENES IN EXTRACTS

5.1 THC (Tetrahydrocannabinol)

Definition:

Tetrahydrocannabinol (THC) is one of the primary cannabinoids found in the cannabis plant. It is the psychoactive compound responsible for the euphoric "high" or altered state of consciousness that is commonly associated with cannabis use.

Chemical Structure:

THC has a complex chemical structure with a bicyclic core (containing two rings) and a side chain. Its full name is $(-)$-trans-Δ^9-tetrahydrocannabinol.

Effects:

THC interacts with the endocannabinoid system (ECS) in the human body, particularly with CB1 receptors located in the brain and central nervous system. This interaction leads to various physiological and psychological effects, including:

1. Euphoria: THC is known for its mood-altering effects, often inducing feelings of euphoria and happiness.

2. Relaxation: It can produce a sense of relaxation and calmness.

3. Altered Perception: THC can affect sensory perception, leading to changes in how individuals perceive time, space, and their surroundings.

4. Increased Appetite: Commonly known as the "munchies," THC can stimulate appetite.

5. Pain Relief: THC has analgesic properties and is used for its pain-relieving effects.

6. Anti-Nausea: THC can help alleviate nausea and vomiting, making it valuable in certain medical treatments.

Medical Uses:

Beyond its recreational use, THC has shown potential therapeutic applications. Medical cannabis formulations containing THC, either alone or in combination with other cannabinoids, are used for:

1. Chronic Pain Management: THC can be effective in managing chronic pain conditions.

2. Nausea and Vomiting: Particularly in cancer patients undergoing chemotherapy.

3. Appetite Stimulation: Beneficial for individuals with appetite loss due to medical conditions.

4. Muscle Spasticity: It may help alleviate muscle spasms and spasticity in conditions such as multiple sclerosis.

5. Glaucoma: THC has been investigated for its potential to reduce intraocular pressure in glaucoma patients.

Different Forms of THC:

1. Delta-9-THC: The most well-known and abundant form of THC in the cannabis plant, responsible for the plant's psychoactive effects.

2. Delta-8-THC: A less common form that is also psychoactive but generally less potent than delta-9-THC.

Metabolism and Elimination:

After consumption, THC is metabolized in the liver, where it transforms into various metabolites, including 11-hydroxy-THC, which is more potent than THC itself. The metabolites are then excreted primarily through urine.

Methods of Consumption:

THC can be consumed in various forms, including:

1. Smoking: Inhaling the smoke from burning cannabis flowers is one of the most traditional methods.

2. Vaporization: Heating cannabis at a lower temperature to produce vapor for inhalation, considered a safer alternative to smoking.

3. Edibles: Cannabis-infused products like brownies, gummies, or beverages provide an alternative to smoking.

4. Tinctures: Liquid extracts of cannabis, often placed under the tongue for sublingual absorption.

5. Topicals: Creams, balms, or patches infused with THC for localized relief without psychoactive effects.

Legality:

The legal status of THC varies globally and regionally. Some places have legalized cannabis for medicinal and/or recreational use, while others maintain strict regulations or prohibition.

Side Effects:

Common side effects of THC consumption include dry mouth, red eyes, impaired coordination, increased heart rate, and short-term memory impairment. High doses may lead to anxiety, paranoia, or hallucinations in some individuals.

It's important for individuals using cannabis, especially products high in THC, to be aware of their local laws, consume responsibly, and be mindful of their own tolerance and susceptibility to potential side effects. Additionally, the therapeutic uses of THC should be approached under the guidance of a healthcare professional.

5.2 CBD (Cannabidiol)

Cannabidiol (CBD) is a natural compound found in the cannabis plant. It belongs to a class of substances known as cannabinoids. Unlike THC (tetrahydrocannabinol), another well-known cannabinoid, CBD is non-psychoactive, meaning it doesn't produce a "high" or altered state of consciousness.

Chemical Structure:

CBD has a chemical structure with a pentyl side chain and two rings. Its full name is 2-[(1R,6R)-3-methyl-6-(1-methylethenyl)-2-cyclohexen-1-yl]-5-pentyl-1,3-benzenediol.

Effects:

While CBD doesn't produce the euphoric effects associated with THC, it interacts with the endocannabinoid system (ECS) in the human body. The ECS plays a role in regulating various physiological processes, and CBD's interactions with it can lead to various effects, including:

1. Anti-Inflammatory: CBD has shown anti-inflammatory properties, making it potentially useful in managing inflammation-related conditions.

2. Analgesic (Pain Relief): CBD may have analgesic effects, contributing to its use in managing various types of pain.

3. Anxiolytic (Anxiety Reduction): CBD has been studied for its potential to reduce anxiety and stress.

4. Antipsychotic: CBD may have antipsychotic properties, and research has explored its use in conditions like schizophrenia.

5. Anti-Seizure: Epidiolex, a CBD-based medication, is approved for the treatment of certain types of epilepsy.

6. Neuroprotective: Some studies suggest that CBD may have neuroprotective effects, potentially beneficial for conditions like neurodegenerative diseases.

Medical Uses:

CBD has gained attention for its potential therapeutic applications, and research is ongoing. Some of the medical uses and areas of interest include:

1. Epilepsy: CBD has shown efficacy in reducing seizures in certain forms of epilepsy, leading to the approval of Epidiolex for this purpose.

2. Chronic Pain: CBD has been studied for its potential role in managing chronic pain conditions.

3. Anxiety and Depression: Some research suggests that CBD may be beneficial in reducing symptoms of anxiety and depression.

4. Inflammatory Conditions: CBD's anti-inflammatory properties may be useful in conditions involving inflammation, such as arthritis.

5. Sleep Disorders: CBD has been explored for its potential to improve sleep in individuals with insomnia or other sleep disorders.

Methods of Consumption:

CBD is available in various forms, and the method of consumption can affect its onset time and duration of effects. Common methods include:

1. Oil/Tinctures: Liquid extracts of CBD that can be taken sublingually (under the tongue) for faster absorption.

2. Capsules: Pre-measured doses of CBD in capsule form for easy and precise consumption.

3. Edibles: CBD-infused products like gummies or beverages provide an alternative to sublingual administration.

4. Topicals: Creams, balms, or patches infused with CBD for localized relief without systemic effects.

5. Vaporization: Inhaling vaporized CBD using a vaporizer for faster onset of effects.

Legality:

The legal status of CBD varies globally and regionally. In many places, CBD derived from industrial hemp with low THC content is legal, while CBD from marijuana may be subject to stricter regulations.

Considerations:

1. Dosage: CBD dosage can vary based on factors such as the individual's weight, the condition being treated, and the form of CBD consumed.

2. Quality: Choose reputable sources for CBD products to ensure product safety and efficacy.

3. Interactions: CBD can interact with certain medications, and individuals should consult with a healthcare professional, especially if they are taking other medications.

4. Full-Spectrum vs. Isolate: Full-spectrum CBD products contain a range of cannabinoids, terpenes, and other compounds from the cannabis plant, potentially enhancing the "entourage effect." CBD isolate is pure CBD without other cannabis compounds.

CBD is generally well-tolerated, but individual responses may vary. It's advisable to approach CBD use with awareness of local regulations, responsible consumption practices, and consideration of individual health factors.

5.3 Other Cannabinoids

In addition to THC and CBD, the cannabis plant contains numerous other cannabinoids, each with its own potential effects and therapeutic properties. Here are some notable cannabinoids found in cannabis:

1. CBG (Cannabigerol):

- Often referred to as the "stem cell" cannabinoid, CBG is a precursor to other cannabinoids. It is usually found in lower concentrations than THC or CBD.
- Potential therapeutic effects include anti-inflammatory, anti-bacterial, and neuroprotective properties.

2. CBC (Cannabichromene):

- CBC is non-psychoactive and is typically found in higher concentrations in tropical cannabis varieties.
- Research suggests potential anti-inflammatory and anti-depressant effects. It may also contribute to the entourage effect when combined with other cannabinoids.

3. CBN (Cannabinol):

- Formed through the degradation of THC, CBN is mildly psychoactive but less potent than THC.
- Often associated with sedative effects, CBN may have potential as a sleep aid.

4. THCV (Tetrahydrocannabivarin):

- THCV is similar to THC but produces different effects at higher doses. It may act as an antagonist to some of the effects of THC.
- Research suggests potential appetite-suppressant and anti-convulsant properties.

5. CBDV (Cannabidivarin):

- CBDV is structurally similar to CBD but has its own distinct properties.
- Some studies indicate potential anti-epileptic effects, making it an area of interest in epilepsy research.

6. Delta-8-THC (Delta-8-Tetrahydrocannabinol):

- Similar to Delta-9-THC, but with a different arrangement of atoms. It is psychoactive but generally less potent than Delta-9-THC.
- Delta-8-THC is gaining popularity as a milder alternative to Delta-9-THC.

7. CBDA (Cannabidiolic Acid):

- The acidic precursor to CBD, CBDA is converted to CBD through decarboxylation (heating).
- Research suggests anti-inflammatory and anti-nausea properties.

8. THCA (Tetrahydrocannabinolic Acid):

- THCA is the acidic precursor to THC and is non-psychoactive until heated (decarboxylation).
- Commonly found in raw cannabis, THCA may have anti-inflammatory and neuroprotective effects.

9. CBN (Cannabinodiol):

- CBN is a degradation product of THC, often forming as cannabis ages.
- Some studies suggest potential anti-bacterial and anti-convulsant properties.

10. CBGA (Cannabigerolic Acid):

- CBGA is the precursor to CBG and other cannabinoids. It plays a key role in the biosynthesis of various cannabinoids.
- Research on CBGA is ongoing, but it is considered a crucial building block for other cannabinoids.

The interaction of these cannabinoids, along with terpenes and other compounds, is known as the "entourage effect." This concept suggests that the combined effects of all cannabis compounds working together may be more beneficial than the effects of individual compounds in isolation. As research continues, a better understanding of each cannabinoid's unique properties and potential benefits will likely emerge.

5.4 Terpenes and Their Role

Terpenes are aromatic compounds found in various plants, including the cannabis plant. These organic compounds contribute to the distinct flavors and aromas of different cannabis strains and play a role in the overall effects of the plant. In addition to cannabis, terpenes are present in fruits, flowers, and herbs, providing them with their characteristic scents.

Common Cannabis Terpenes:

1. Myrcene:

- Aroma: Earthy, musky, herbal.

- Effects: Sedative, relaxing.

- Found In: Mangoes, hops, thyme.

2. Limonene:

- Aroma: Citrus, lemon.

- Effects: Uplifting, mood-enhancing.

- Found In: Citrus fruits, juniper, peppermint.

3. Pinene:

- Aroma: Pine, earthy.

- Effects: Alertness, memory retention.

- Found In: Pine needles, rosemary, basil.

4. Caryophyllene:

   - Aroma: Spicy, peppery.

   - Effects: Anti-inflammatory, calming.

   - Found In: Black pepper, cloves, cinnamon.

5. Linalool:

   - Aroma: Floral, lavender.

   - Effects: Relaxing, anti-anxiety.

   - Found In: Lavender, coriander, rosewood.

6. Humulene:

   - Aroma: Woody, earthy.

   - Effects: Appetite suppressant.

   - Found In: Hops, sage, ginseng.

7. Terpinolene:

   - Aroma: Floral, herbal, fruity.

   - Effects: Energizing, anti-anxiety.

   - Found In: Apples, cumin, lilacs.

8. Ocimene:

- Aroma: Sweet, citrus, tropical.

- Effects: Energizing, anti-inflammatory.

- Found In: Mint, parsley, orchids.

Role of Terpenes:

1. Entourage Effect:

- Terpenes, along with cannabinoids, contribute to the entourage effect, where the combined compounds enhance each other's effects. The presence of specific terpenes can modify or amplify the effects of cannabinoids like THC and CBD.

2. Aroma and Flavor:

- Terpenes are responsible for the diverse scents and flavors of different cannabis strains. The aromatic profile can range from citrus and pine to floral and spicy, influencing the overall user experience.

3. Effects and Therapeutic Properties:

- Terpenes are believed to have therapeutic properties. For example, myrcene may contribute to the relaxing effects of some strains, while limonene may have mood-enhancing properties. These properties can vary based on the specific combination of terpenes in a given strain.

4. Modulation of Cannabinoid Reception:

- Some terpenes may interact with cannabinoid receptors and neurotransmitter systems, influencing the way cannabinoids bind to receptors. This modulation can impact the overall effects of cannabis.

5. Differentiation of Strains:

- Terpene profiles are often used to differentiate cannabis strains. For example, strains with high levels of myrcene may be labeled as indicas, associated with sedative effects, while strains with limonene may be labeled as sativas, associated with uplifting effects.

Terpene Extraction:

- Terpenes can be extracted from cannabis using various methods, such as steam distillation or hydrodistillation. These extracted terpenes can be reintroduced into cannabis products, contributing to the preservation of the strain's original aroma and potential entourage effects.

Considerations:

- Understanding the terpene profile of a cannabis strain can provide users with insights into the potential effects and flavors they might experience.
- Personal preferences for specific terpene profiles may guide individuals in selecting strains that suit their desired experiences.
- The interaction between terpenes and cannabinoids is a complex and dynamic aspect of the cannabis plant, and ongoing research continues to unveil the intricacies of these interactions.

In summary, terpenes play a crucial role in shaping the unique characteristics of each cannabis strain, influencing both the sensory experience and the potential therapeutic effects.

6. METHODS OF CONSUMPTION

6.1 Smoking Cannabis: Methods, Effects and Considerations

1. Joint:

- A joint is a cannabis cigarette made by rolling ground cannabis flower in rolling papers.
- It is a traditional and straightforward method of smoking.

2. Blunt:

- Similar to a joint, a blunt is made by rolling cannabis in a cigar wrapper or hollowed-out cigar.
- Blunts are typically larger than joints and can contain more cannabis.

3. Pipe:

- A pipe is a small, portable device with a bowl for holding cannabis flower. Users inhale through a mouthpiece.
- Pipes come in various materials, including glass, metal, and wood.

4. Bong (Water Pipe):

- A bong is a water filtration device that cools and filters smoke before inhalation.
- Users light the cannabis in a bowl, and the smoke passes through water before reaching the mouthpiece.

5. Vaporizer:

- Vaporizers heat cannabis to a temperature that releases cannabinoids and terpenes without combustion.
- Vaporization is considered a less harmful alternative to smoking as it produces fewer harmful byproducts.

Effects of Smoking Cannabis:

1. Rapid Onset:

- Smoking provides one of the quickest ways to feel the effects of cannabis, with onset occurring within minutes.

2. Short Duration:

- The effects of smoking typically peak within 30 minutes to an hour and gradually diminish over a few hours.

3. Bioavailability:

- Smoking delivers cannabinoids directly into the bloodstream through the lungs, resulting in high bioavailability.

4. Characteristics of High:

- The "high" from smoking cannabis is often characterized by euphoria, relaxation, altered sensory perception, increased appetite, and heightened creativity.

Considerations for Smoking Cannabis:

1. Dosage Control:

- It can be challenging to control the dosage when smoking, as the effects are felt rapidly, and it's easy to consume more than intended.

2. Respiratory Health:

- Smoking involves inhaling combusted plant material, which may pose respiratory risks. Long-term smoking can irritate the lungs and may contribute to respiratory issues.

3. Secondhand Smoke:

- Secondhand smoke from cannabis can affect non-smokers in proximity. It's essential to be mindful of the environment when smoking.

4. Tolerance and Dependency:

- Regular smoking can lead to the development of tolerance, where higher doses are needed to achieve the same effects. Some individuals may also develop a psychological dependency.

5. Legality:

- Smoking cannabis may be subject to legal restrictions depending on the jurisdiction. It's crucial to be aware of and adhere to local laws.

6. Smoking Alternatives:

- Individuals concerned about the potential health risks of smoking may explore alternative methods of consumption, such as vaporization or edibles.

7. Strain Selection:

- Different cannabis strains have distinct effects and terpene profiles. Users may choose strains based on their desired experiences.

8. Setting and Comfort:

- The environment in which cannabis is smoked can impact the overall experience. Being in a comfortable and familiar setting can enhance enjoyment.

Health Considerations:

- While some studies suggest a link between long-term cannabis smoking and respiratory issues, more research is needed to fully understand the extent of these risks.

- Vaporization is considered a less harmful method of consumption as it avoids combustion, reducing exposure to harmful byproducts.

6.2 Vaporizing

Vaporizing, or vaping, is a method of cannabis consumption that involves heating cannabis material to a temperature that releases cannabinoids and terpenes in the form of vapor, without combustion. Vaporization is considered a less harmful alternative to smoking, as it avoids the production of many of the harmful byproducts associated with combustion.

Components of a Vaporizer:

1. Heating Element:

- The heating element is responsible for heating the cannabis material to the desired temperature. Common types include conduction (direct contact with the heating element) and convection (hot air passing through the material).

2. Chamber:

- The chamber holds the cannabis material and is the space where vaporization occurs. It can be made of materials like ceramic, stainless steel, or quartz.

3. Battery:

- Vaporizers are powered by batteries, providing the energy needed to heat the element. Batteries can be rechargeable or replaceable.

4. Temperature Control:

- Some vaporizers allow users to control the temperature at which the cannabis is heated, providing flexibility in the vaporization experience.

Advantages of Vaporizing:

1. Reduced Harmful Byproducts:

- Vaporization occurs at a lower temperature than combustion, resulting in the release of vapor without the production of many of the harmful substances associated with smoking.

2. Preservation of Flavor and Aroma:

- Vaporization preserves the flavors and aromas of cannabis more effectively than combustion, allowing users to experience the full terpene profile.

3. Controlled Dosage:

- Vaporizers allow for more precise control over dosage, as users can monitor the amount of material loaded and adjust temperature settings.

4. Quick Onset:

- Vaporization provides a rapid onset of effects, similar to smoking, as the vaporized cannabinoids are quickly absorbed into the bloodstream through the lungs.

5. Portability and Discreetness:

- Many vaporizers are portable and discreet, making them convenient for on-the-go use.

Effects of Vaporizing Cannabis:

1. Similar to Smoking:

- The effects of vaporizing cannabis are similar to smoking, including a rapid onset of euphoria, relaxation, altered sensory perception, and increased appetite.

2. Controlled and Precise:

- Vaporizing allows for a more controlled and precise experience, as users can adjust temperature settings to influence the composition of vapor.

3. Cleaner Experience:

- Users often report a cleaner and smoother experience when vaporizing compared to smoking.

Considerations for Vaporizing Cannabis:

1. Temperature Settings:

- Different cannabinoids and terpenes vaporize at different temperatures. Experimenting with temperature settings can influence the overall experience.

2. Maintenance:

- Regular cleaning and maintenance of the vaporizer are essential to ensure optimal performance and prevent the buildup of residue.

3. Material Quality:

- The quality of the cannabis material used in the vaporizer can significantly impact the vaporization experience. High-quality, well-cured cannabis generally produces better results.

4. Legal Considerations:

- While vaporizing is often considered a discreet method of consumption, users should be aware of and adhere to local laws and regulations regarding cannabis use.

5. Health Considerations:

- While vaporizing is generally considered a safer option than smoking, more research is needed to fully understand the long-term health implications.

.

6.3 Edibles

Edibles are food and beverage products infused with cannabis extracts, such as THC (tetrahydrocannabinol) or CBD (cannabidiol). They offer an alternative method of cannabis consumption to smoking or vaporization and are known for their discreet nature and longer-lasting effects.

Types of Edibles:

1. Baked Goods:

- Brownies, cookies, cakes, and muffins are common baked goods infused with cannabis extracts. They often have a rich and dense texture.

2. Candies:

- Gummies, chocolates, hard candies, and lollipops are popular choices. They provide a sweet and convenient way to consume cannabis.

3. Beverages:

- Cannabis-infused beverages include teas, coffees, sodas, and fruit juices. These beverages offer a refreshing and discreet option.

4. Capsules:

- Cannabis oil or powder is encapsulated, providing a measured and controlled dose. Capsules are tasteless and easy to incorporate into a daily routine.

5. Tinctures:

- Liquid cannabis extracts that can be consumed sublingually (under the tongue) or added to food and beverages. Tinctures allow for precise dosage control.

6. Snack Foods:

- Chips, pretzels, popcorn, and other snack items can be infused with cannabis. They offer a savory alternative to sweet edibles.

Effects and Onset:

1. Onset Time:

- The onset of effects from edibles is typically slower compared to smoking or vaporizing. It can take anywhere from 30 minutes to 2 hours for effects to be felt, depending on factors like metabolism and the individual's digestive system.

2. Duration of Effects:

- Edibles often provide a longer-lasting high compared to inhalation methods. The effects can last anywhere from 4 to 12 hours.

3. Intensity:

- Edibles can produce a more intense and sedative high compared to smoking or vaporizing, especially at higher doses.

Dosage Considerations:

1. Start Low and Go Slow:

- It's recommended to start with a low dosage, especially for individuals new to edibles. The effects can be potent, and it's essential to allow time for onset before consuming more.

2. Labeling and Packaging:

- Edibles are often labeled with the total cannabinoid content (e.g., THC or CBD) and the serving size. Paying attention to these details helps in controlling dosage.

3. Individual Sensitivity:

- Sensitivity to edibles can vary among individuals. Factors such as body weight, metabolism, and tolerance levels can influence the response to a given dose.

Considerations for Safe Consumption:

1. Patience:

- Due to the slower onset time, it's crucial to be patient and avoid consuming additional doses too quickly.

2. Legal Compliance:

- Adherence to local laws and regulations regarding the purchase, possession, and consumption of cannabis-infused edibles is essential.

3. Safe Storage:

- Store edibles securely and out of reach of children and pets. Packaging should be child-resistant, and clear labeling is important.

4. Awareness of Surroundings:

- The long-lasting effects of edibles can impact activities and cognitive function. It's important to consume edibles in a safe and familiar environment.

Potential Health Risks:

1. Overconsumption:

- Overconsumption of edibles can lead to discomfort, anxiety, and an overly intense high. Starting with a low dose and waiting before consuming more can help avoid this.

2. Delayed Effects:

- The delayed onset of effects may lead some individuals to consume more, thinking the initial dose was ineffective. This can result in unintended and potent effects.

3. Interaction with Medications:

- Individuals taking medications should consult with a healthcare professional before consuming cannabis edibles, as there may be interactions.

6.4 Topicals

Cannabis topicals are products infused with cannabis extracts, such as CBD (cannabidiol) or THC (tetrahydrocannabinol), designed for external application on the skin. These products include creams, balms, lotions, salves, and patches. Unlike edibles or inhaled forms of cannabis, topicals do not produce a psychoactive "high" as the cannabinoids typically do not enter the bloodstream.

How Cannabis Topicals Work:

1. Localized Effects:

- Cannabis topicals are applied directly to the skin, where they interact with the endocannabinoid receptors in the skin's ECS (endocannabinoid system). This interaction is thought to produce localized therapeutic effects without affecting the central nervous system.

2. No Psychoactive Effects:

- The cannabinoids in topicals generally do not penetrate deeply enough to reach the bloodstream, resulting in minimal systemic absorption. This means that even if the topical contains THC, it is unlikely to cause psychoactive effects.

Types of Cannabis Topicals:

1. Creams and Lotions:

- Cannabis-infused creams and lotions are formulated for general skincare and may contain additional ingredients like moisturizers and essential oils.

2. Balms and Salves:

- Balms and salves are thicker in consistency and are often used for targeted relief. They may contain a combination of cannabinoids, terpenes, and other therapeutic ingredients.

3. Patches:

- Transdermal patches are adhesive patches infused with cannabinoids. They are designed to deliver a controlled dose of cannabinoids through the skin over an extended period.

4. Roll-Ons:

- Roll-on topicals typically come in a bottle with a rollerball applicator, making them easy to apply. They are convenient for targeted relief and may include additional ingredients like menthol.

5. Pain Patches:

- These are adhesive patches infused with cannabinoids and other pain-relieving ingredients. They are designed specifically for addressing localized pain.

Common Uses and Benefits:

1. Pain Relief:

- Cannabis topicals are often used to alleviate localized pain, including muscle soreness, joint pain, and neuropathic pain.

2. Anti-Inflammatory Effects:

- The anti-inflammatory properties of cannabinoids may help reduce inflammation associated with conditions like arthritis and dermatitis.

3. Skin Conditions:

- Topicals may provide relief for skin conditions such as eczema, psoriasis, and acne due to their anti-inflammatory and moisturizing properties.

4. Localized Relaxation:

- Cannabis-infused topicals may promote localized relaxation and tension relief when applied to areas of the body experiencing stress or tension.

5. Muscle Recovery:

- Athletes and individuals engaging in physical activities may use topicals to aid in muscle recovery and alleviate post-exercise soreness.

Considerations for Using Cannabis Topicals:

1. Application:

- Follow the product's instructions for application. Topicals are generally applied directly to the affected area of the skin.

2. Dosage:

- While it's challenging to overdose on topicals, it's advisable to start with a small amount and monitor the effects.

3. Patch Testing:

- Perform a patch test on a small area of skin to check for any adverse reactions before applying a larger amount.

4. Consistency:

- Consistent use may be necessary to experience the full benefits of cannabis topicals. Results can vary among individuals.

5. Interactions:

- If using other topical medications or skincare products, consider potential interactions. Consult with a healthcare professional if needed.

6. Storage:

- Store cannabis topicals in a cool, dry place and follow any specific storage instructions provided by the manufacturer.

6.5 Dabbing

Dabbing is a method of consuming cannabis concentrates, which are highly potent extracts of cannabinoids such as THC (tetrahydrocannabinol) or CBD (cannabidiol). The term "dab" refers to a small amount of concentrate that is vaporized and inhaled. Dabbing involves the use of specialized tools and equipment, such as a dab rig or vaporizer, to achieve quick and intense effects.

Components of Dabbing:

1. Cannabis Concentrate:

- Dabs are made from cannabis extracts, which can take various forms, including wax, shatter, budder, or oil. These concentrates are rich in cannabinoids and terpenes.

2. Dab Rig:

- A dab rig is a water pipe specifically designed for vaporizing concentrates. It typically includes a water chamber, a nail (heating element), and a dabber (tool for placing the concentrate on the nail).

3. Nail:

- The nail is the part of the dab rig where the concentrate is placed and vaporized. Nails can be made of various materials, such as quartz, titanium, or ceramic.

4. Dabber:

- The dabber is a tool used to place a small amount of concentrate onto the heated nail. It can be made of metal, glass, or other materials.

5. Torch:

- A butane torch is often used to heat the nail to high temperatures quickly. Electric or e-nails are alternatives that eliminate the need for a torch.

Dabbing Process:

1. Preparation:

- Place a small amount of cannabis concentrate (a dab) on the end of the dabber.

2. Heating the Nail:

- Heat the nail with a torch until it reaches the desired temperature. The optimal temperature for vaporization is often lower than that for combustion.

3. Applying the Dab:

- Once the nail is sufficiently heated, use the dabber to apply the concentrate to the hot surface. Vaporization occurs, producing a vapor that is inhaled.

4. Inhalation:

- Inhale the vapor through the mouthpiece of the dab rig. Some rigs may have additional percolators to cool and filter the vapor.

Advantages of Dabbing:

1. Potency:

- Cannabis concentrates are highly potent, containing a high concentration of cannabinoids. Dabbing allows users to experience intense effects quickly.

2. Quick Onset:

- The effects of dabbing are felt almost immediately, providing rapid relief for medical or recreational purposes.

3. Precise Dosage:

- Dabbing allows for precise dosage control, as users can measure the amount of concentrate used in each session.

4. Flavor Profiles:

- Some users appreciate the rich and diverse flavor profiles of different cannabis concentrates, which can include terpenes and other compounds.

Considerations for Dabbing:

1. High Potency:

- Cannabis concentrates are much more potent than traditional flower. Users, especially beginners, should start with small doses to avoid overconsumption.

2. Equipment Maintenance:

- Regular cleaning and maintenance of dabbing equipment are essential to preserve the flavor and efficiency of the dab rig.

3. Temperature Control:

- Controlling the temperature is crucial for a good dabbing experience. High temperatures can lead to combustion, affecting flavor and potentially producing harsher vapor.

4. Safety:

- Dabbing involves the use of a torch or heating element, so safety precautions, such as proper ventilation and fire safety, should be observed.

5. Legal Considerations:

- Cannabis concentrates and dabbing may be subject to specific legal regulations depending on the jurisdiction. Users should be aware of and comply with local laws.

Conclusion:

Dabbing is a method of cannabis consumption appreciated by enthusiasts for its potency and quick onset of effects. While it requires specialized equipment and careful attention to dosage, temperature, and safety, many users find dabbing to be an efficient way to experience the benefits of cannabis concentrates. As with any form of cannabis consumption, responsible and informed use is crucial.

7. DOSAGE AND SAFETY

7.1 Understanding Dosage

Understanding cannabis dosage is essential for achieving a safe and enjoyable experience. The appropriate dosage can vary widely among individuals due to factors such as tolerance, body weight, metabolism, and individual sensitivity. Here are key considerations for understanding cannabis dosage:

1. Start Low and Go Slow:

- This principle is commonly recommended for individuals new to cannabis or a particular product. Begin with a low dose and gradually increase it over time as needed. This approach helps minimize the risk of adverse effects.

2. Individual Tolerance:

- Tolerance to cannabis can develop with regular use, meaning that higher doses may be needed to achieve the same effects. It's important to be mindful of individual tolerance levels.

3. THC and CBD Content:

- The ratio of THC to CBD in a cannabis product significantly influences its effects. THC is psychoactive and produces the "high" associated with cannabis, while CBD is non-psychoactive and may have various therapeutic properties. Understanding the cannabinoid content is crucial for predicting the potential effects of a product.

4. Product Type:

- Different cannabis products (flower, edibles, concentrates, tinctures, etc.) have varying levels of potency. For example, edibles can be more potent and have a longer onset time compared to smoking or vaporizing.

5. Labeling and Packaging:

- Many regulated cannabis products provide information on the packaging, including the total cannabinoid content, serving size, and sometimes recommended dosages. Pay attention to these details to ensure accurate dosing.

6. Route of Administration:

- The method of consumption influences how cannabinoids are absorbed into the body. Inhalation (smoking or vaporizing) generally has a quicker onset, while edibles take longer but may produce longer-lasting effects.

7. Body Weight and Metabolism:

- Body weight and metabolism play a role in how cannabinoids are processed in the body. Individuals with higher body weight may require larger doses to feel the same effects.

8. Health Conditions and Medications:

- Some health conditions and medications can interact with cannabis. Individuals with pre-existing conditions or those taking medications should consult with a healthcare professional before using cannabis.

9. Consistency of Products:

- Consistency is crucial when using cannabis products. Batch variations in potency can occur, so it's advisable to stick with products from reputable sources.

10. Personal Preferences:

- Individual preferences and goals for cannabis use also influence dosage decisions. Some users may prefer lower doses for subtle effects, while others may seek higher doses for more pronounced effects.

11. Observing Effects:

- Pay attention to how your body responds to different doses. If using a new product or trying a different method of consumption, start with a small amount and observe the effects before deciding to increase the dosage.

12. Adverse Effects:

- Be aware of potential adverse effects, such as anxiety, paranoia, or discomfort. If such effects occur, it's advisable to reduce the dosage or discontinue use.

13. Patience:

- Especially with edibles, it's crucial to be patient. The effects may take longer to manifest, and consuming more before the onset can lead to overconsumption.

7.2 Risks and Precautions

Using cannabis, like any substance, comes with certain risks, and it's essential to take precautions to ensure a safe and positive experience. Here are some common risks associated with cannabis use and precautions to consider:

1. Impaired Coordination and Cognition:

- Risk: Cannabis can impair coordination, attention, and reaction time, increasing the risk of accidents, especially when operating vehicles or heavy machinery.
- Precautions: Avoid driving or engaging in activities that require focus and coordination while under the influence of cannabis. Plan for alternative transportation if needed.

2. Psychological Effects:

- Risk: Cannabis use may exacerbate anxiety, paranoia, or other mental health conditions, especially in individuals predisposed to these issues.
- Precautions: If you have a history of mental health issues, consult with a healthcare professional before using cannabis. Start with low doses, and be aware of how cannabis affects your mental state.

3. Overconsumption:

- Risk: Consuming too much cannabis can lead to adverse effects such as anxiety, paranoia, nausea, or vomiting.

- Precautions: Start with low doses, especially if you are a new or infrequent user. Be aware of the potency of the product and give yourself time between doses.

4. Respiratory Risks (Smoking):

- Risk: Smoking cannabis involves inhaling combusted plant material, which can irritate the lungs and potentially lead to respiratory issues.
- Precautions: Consider alternative methods of consumption, such as vaporization or edibles, to reduce respiratory risks. If smoking, use clean and well-maintained equipment.

5. Cardiovascular Effects:

- Risk: Cannabis use can lead to increased heart rate and blood pressure, which may pose risks for individuals with cardiovascular issues.
- Precautions: Individuals with heart conditions should consult with a healthcare professional before using cannabis. Monitor your heart rate and blood pressure, especially if you have concerns.

6. Cognitive Development in Adolescents:

- Risk: Cannabis use during adolescence may impact cognitive development, including memory and learning.
- Precautions: Delay cannabis use until the brain is fully developed, typically in the mid-20s. If you are a parent or caregiver, educate adolescents about the potential risks.

7. Dependency and Addiction:

- Risk: Regular use of cannabis can lead to the development of tolerance and dependency in some individuals.
- Precautions: Use cannabis responsibly and avoid habitual or excessive use. If you suspect dependency issues, seek support from healthcare professionals or addiction counselors.

8. Interaction with Medications:

- Risk: Cannabis may interact with certain medications, potentially affecting their efficacy or causing adverse effects.
- Precautions: Consult with a healthcare professional before using cannabis, especially if you are taking prescription medications. Be transparent about your cannabis use to receive appropriate medical guidance.

9. Legal Considerations:

- Risk: Cannabis laws vary widely among jurisdictions, and using or possessing cannabis may be illegal in some places.
- Precautions: Be aware of the legal status of cannabis in your location. Adhere to local laws and regulations to avoid legal consequences.

10. Pregnancy and Breastfeeding:

- Risk: Cannabis use during pregnancy and breastfeeding may have potential risks for the developing fetus or infant.
- Precautions: Pregnant and breastfeeding individuals should consult with healthcare professionals and avoid cannabis use during these periods.

11. Edible Caution:

- Risk: Edibles can lead to overconsumption and delayed onset of effects, increasing the risk of accidental overuse.
- Precautions: Start with low doses when consuming edibles. Be patient, as the effects may take longer to manifest compared to smoking or vaporizing.

7.3 Responsible Use

Responsible cannabis use involves making informed and mindful choices to ensure a positive and safe experience. Whether using cannabis for recreational or medical purposes, the following guidelines can help promote responsible use:

1. Know the Laws:

- Understand and adhere to the cannabis laws and regulations in your jurisdiction. This includes rules around possession, cultivation, and consumption.

2. Understand the Product:

- Be aware of the potency, cannabinoid content (e.g., THC and CBD), and potential effects of the cannabis product you are using. Read product labels and follow recommended dosage guidelines.

3. Start Low and Go Slow:

- If you are new to cannabis or trying a new product, start with a low dose. Gradually increase the dosage as needed, allowing time between doses to assess effects.

4. Choose the Right Environment:

- Consume cannabis in a comfortable and familiar setting. Consider factors such as your mood, the presence of others, and the overall environment to ensure a positive experience.

5. Avoid Mixing with Other Substances:

- Combining cannabis with alcohol or other substances can intensify the effects and increase the risk of adverse reactions. Consume cannabis in isolation to better understand its effects on your body.

6. Monitor Frequency of Use:

- Be mindful of how often you use cannabis. Regular, heavy use may lead to tolerance and potential dependence. Consider periods of abstinence to maintain a healthy relationship with the substance.

7. Respect Personal Limits:

- Understand your own tolerance and set personal limits for cannabis use. Avoid peer pressure and only consume what you feel comfortable with.

8. Consider Your Health:

- If you have pre-existing health conditions or are taking medications, consult with a healthcare professional before using cannabis. Be transparent about your cannabis use during medical consultations.

9. Be Mindful of Others:

- Respect the rights and boundaries of others, especially in shared spaces. Avoid exposing non-consenting individuals to secondhand smoke or vapor.

10. Store Cannabis Securely:

- Keep cannabis products, especially edibles, out of reach of children and pets. Store them securely to prevent accidental consumption.

11. Educate Yourself:

- Stay informed about cannabis, including its effects, potential risks, and new developments in the field. Knowledgeable consumers are better equipped to make responsible choices.

12. Plan Ahead:

- If using cannabis in social settings, plan ahead for transportation and avoid driving under the influence.

Arrange for a designated driver, public transportation, or rideshare services.

13. Be Cautious with Edibles:

- Edibles can have delayed onset times and produce potent effects. Start with a low dose, be patient, and avoid consuming additional servings too quickly.

14. Seek Support if Needed:

- If you find that your cannabis use is impacting your daily life, mental health, or relationships, consider seeking support from healthcare professionals or addiction counselors.

15. Promote Safe Consumption Methods:

- Choose consumption methods that align with your health goals. For example, consider vaporization or edibles as alternatives to smoking to reduce respiratory risks.

In summary, responsible cannabis use involves a combination of education, self-awareness, and consideration for others. By following these guidelines and being mindful of your choices, you can contribute to a positive and safe cannabis experience for yourself and those around you.

8. CHOOSING THE RIGHT EXTRACT

8.1 Personal Preferences

Personal preferences in cannabis consumption can vary widely among individuals, and understanding these preferences is crucial for a positive and enjoyable experience. Here are some factors that contribute to personal preferences in cannabis use:

1. Desired Effects:

- Individuals may have different goals when using cannabis. Some may seek relaxation, stress relief, or pain management, while others may be interested in creativity, focus, or socialization. Understanding your desired effects helps guide product selection and dosage.

2. Tolerance Levels:

- Tolerance to cannabis varies among individuals. Some people may be more sensitive to cannabinoids, while others may require higher doses to feel the same effects. Knowing your tolerance helps with dosage control.

3. Product Type:

- Preferences for cannabis products can vary. Some individuals may prefer smoking or vaporizing flower for its immediate effects, while others may opt for edibles for a longer-lasting experience. Cannabis concentrates and topicals offer additional options.

4. Flavor and Aroma:

- The flavor and aroma of cannabis can significantly influence preferences. Different strains and products have distinct terpene profiles, contributing to their unique scents and tastes. Some individuals may prefer fruity, floral, or earthy notes.

5. Consumption Method:

- The method of consumption can impact the overall experience. Some users prefer the ritual of rolling and smoking a joint, while others may appreciate the convenience and discretion of vaporization. Edibles and tinctures offer alternative methods.

6. Social or Solo Use:

- Personal preferences may be influenced by whether cannabis is consumed socially or in solitude. Some individuals enjoy the communal aspect of sharing a joint, while others prefer the introspective experience of consuming alone.

7. Cannabinoid Ratio:

   - The ratio of cannabinoids, such as THC to CBD, can influence the overall effects. Individuals seeking a psychoactive "high" may prefer higher THC content, while those prioritizing relaxation or therapeutic effects may choose products with balanced or higher CBD content.

8. Strain Preferences:

   - Cannabis strains have different characteristics, and individuals may have preferences based on their effects. Sativa strains are often associated with energizing effects, indicas with relaxation, and hybrids with a combination of both.

9. Medical or Recreational Use:

   - The purpose of cannabis use, whether for medical or recreational reasons, can shape preferences. Medical users may prioritize products with specific therapeutic properties, while recreational users may focus on enjoyment and relaxation.

10. Product Potency:

   - Some individuals prefer products with higher potency for more pronounced effects, while others may opt for lower-potency options to control their experience more precisely.

11. Setting and Atmosphere:

- The environment in which cannabis is consumed can influence preferences. Whether in a natural setting, at home, or in a social setting, the atmosphere plays a role in the overall experience.

12. Cultural and Social Influences:

- Cultural and social factors can shape preferences. Cultural backgrounds, regional norms, and social circles may influence the types of products and consumption methods individuals are exposed to and comfortable with.

Understanding and respecting personal preferences in cannabis use contribute to a more positive and tailored experience. Experimenting with different strains, products, and consumption methods allows individuals to discover what works best for them and aligns with their goals and preferences. Additionally, staying informed about the latest developments in the cannabis industry can open up new possibilities for exploration.

8.2 Medical Considerations

When considering cannabis for medical purposes, it's important to approach its use with careful consideration, especially if you have pre-existing health conditions or are taking medications. Here are key medical considerations for using cannabis:

1. Consult with a Healthcare Professional:

- Before using cannabis for medical reasons, consult with a healthcare professional, preferably one with expertise in medical cannabis. They can provide personalized guidance based on your health history and needs.

2. Disclose Cannabis Use to Healthcare Providers:

- Be open and transparent with your healthcare providers about your cannabis use. This information is crucial for them to make informed decisions about your overall health and potential interactions with medications.

3. Understand Potential Interactions:

- Cannabis may interact with certain medications, either enhancing or diminishing their effects. Understanding potential interactions is crucial to avoid adverse effects or reduced medication efficacy.

4. Consider Different Consumption Methods:

- Different methods of cannabis consumption may have varying effects on the body. For example, vaporization or tinctures may be preferred over smoking for individuals with respiratory concerns. Discuss with your healthcare provider to determine the most suitable method for your needs.

5. Focus on Cannabinoid Ratios:

- Consider the cannabinoid profile of cannabis products, especially the ratio of THC (tetrahydrocannabinol) to CBD (cannabidiol). CBD is non-psychoactive and may have therapeutic properties without the euphoric effects associated with THC.

6. Target Specific Symptoms:

- Cannabis may be used to target specific symptoms associated with various medical conditions. For example, it may be helpful for pain management, nausea, anxiety, or sleep disturbances. Tailor your cannabis use to address your specific symptoms.

7. Start with Low Doses:

- If you are new to medical cannabis or trying a new product, start with a low dose and gradually titrate upward. This approach helps to assess your tolerance and minimize the risk of adverse effects.

8. Be Aware of Potential Risks:

- Understand the potential risks associated with cannabis use, especially if you have a history of mental health issues, cardiovascular concerns, or other health conditions. Consult with your healthcare provider to weigh the potential benefits against risks.

9. Monitor Effects and Adjust Dosage:

- Regularly monitor the effects of cannabis on your symptoms and adjust the dosage as needed. Keep a log of your cannabis use and its impact on your health to share with your healthcare provider.

10. Consider CBD-Only Products:

- If avoiding the psychoactive effects of THC is a priority, consider using CBD-only products. These products contain no or minimal THC and may still offer therapeutic benefits.

11. Legal Considerations:

- Be aware of the legal status of medical cannabis in your jurisdiction. Understand the regulations regarding medical cannabis use, including obtaining a medical cannabis card if required.

12. Pregnancy and Breastfeeding:

- Pregnant and breastfeeding individuals should exercise caution with cannabis use, as it may have potential risks for the developing fetus or infant. Consult with healthcare professionals for guidance.

13. Stay Informed:

- Stay informed about the latest research and developments in the field of medical cannabis. New products, delivery methods, and formulations are continually being explored, and staying informed allows you to make educated decisions.

14. Quality of Cannabis Products:

- Consider the quality and source of the cannabis products you use. Choose products from reputable sources that adhere to quality and safety standards.

In summary, approaching medical cannabis use with a thoughtful and informed mindset is essential. Collaboration with healthcare professionals, careful consideration of individual health factors, and ongoing monitoring of effects contribute to a responsible and potentially beneficial use of cannabis for medical purposes.

8.3 Legal Considerations

Legal considerations regarding cannabis use vary widely depending on the jurisdiction and local laws. It's crucial to be aware of and adhere to the legal regulations surrounding cannabis in your specific location. Here are some general points to consider:

1. Know Your Local Laws:

- Cannabis laws differ significantly from country to country, and even within regions of a country. Research and understand the specific regulations governing cannabis use, possession, cultivation, and distribution in your area.

2. Medical vs. Recreational Use:

- Different jurisdictions may have separate regulations for medical and recreational cannabis use. Ensure that you understand the distinctions and requirements for each category.

3. Medical Cannabis Programs:

- In some regions, medical cannabis may be legal for qualifying patients under specific conditions. If you are considering medical cannabis, check if your jurisdiction has a medical cannabis program, and if so, follow the necessary procedures to enroll.

4. Cannabis Possession Limits:

- Know the legal limits for cannabis possession in your area. These limits can vary, and exceeding them may result in legal consequences.

5. Age Restrictions:

- Many jurisdictions have age restrictions for cannabis use, similar to those for alcohol. Be aware of the legal age for cannabis consumption in your area and adhere to it.

6. Cultivation Regulations:

- If you are interested in growing cannabis for personal use, be aware of the regulations and limitations on cultivation. Some areas allow limited home cultivation, while others may prohibit it entirely.

7. Distribution and Sales:

- Understand the rules governing the distribution and sale of cannabis. In some places, only licensed dispensaries are permitted to sell cannabis products. Unauthorized sales may lead to legal consequences.

8. Public vs. Private Consumption:

- Laws regarding public cannabis consumption vary. Some jurisdictions permit private use but prohibit public consumption. Familiarize yourself with the rules regarding where you can and cannot consume cannabis.

9. Driving Under the Influence:

- Driving under the influence of cannabis is illegal in most places. Be aware of the legal limits for THC in your system and avoid driving if you are impaired.

10. Federal vs. State/Provincial Laws:

- In some countries, cannabis laws may vary between federal and state or provincial levels. For example, cannabis may be legal at the state level but illegal at the federal level. Understand the hierarchy of laws in your jurisdiction.

11. Employment Considerations:

- Some employers have policies regarding cannabis use, even in areas where it is legal. Understand your workplace policies to avoid any potential conflicts.

12. Traveling with Cannabis:

- Cannabis possession laws can differ when crossing borders or traveling between regions. Research the laws of your destination to avoid legal issues.

13. Legalization Changes:

- Cannabis laws are subject to change. Stay informed about any updates or changes to the legal status of cannabis in your area.

14. Legal Consultation:

- If you have specific legal questions or concerns, consider consulting with a legal professional who specializes in cannabis law to receive personalized advice.

In summary, staying informed about the legal landscape of cannabis in your jurisdiction is crucial for responsible and lawful consumption. Ignorance of the law is not a valid defense, so take the time to research and understand the specific regulations that apply to your situation. If in doubt, seek legal advice to ensure that you are in compliance with local laws.

9. STORAGE AND PRESERVATION

9.1 Best Practices for Storing Extracts

Proper storage of cannabis extracts is essential to maintain their potency, flavor, and overall quality. Here are some best practices for storing extracts:

1. Cool and Dark Environment:

- Store cannabis extracts in a cool and dark environment to minimize exposure to light and heat. Light and heat can degrade cannabinoids and terpenes, leading to a loss of potency and flavor.

2. Airtight Containers:

- Use airtight containers to prevent exposure to air, which can oxidize the extracts and degrade their quality over time. Containers with a silicone lining can be beneficial in preventing terpene loss.

3. Avoid Temperature Fluctuations:

- Avoid temperature fluctuations, as extreme changes in temperature can affect the consistency of extracts and lead to separation. Keep extracts in a consistently cool environment.

4. Refrigeration or Freezing (Depending on Consistency):

- For certain types of extracts, such as concentrates like shatter or wax, refrigeration or freezing can help maintain their stability. However, avoid freezing extracts with high moisture content, as this can lead to the formation of ice crystals.

5. Keep Away from Light:

- Light can degrade cannabinoids and terpenes. Store extracts in opaque containers or keep them in a dark place to protect them from exposure to light.

6. Avoid Humidity:

- Excessive humidity can lead to the growth of mold, affecting the quality and safety of cannabis extracts. Keep extracts in a low-humidity environment to prevent moisture-related issues.

7. Separate Flavors and Strains:

- If storing multiple extracts with distinct flavors and strains, consider keeping them in separate containers to prevent cross-contamination of aromas and flavors.

8. Labeling:

- Clearly label your extracts with information such as the strain, extraction date, and any other relevant details. This helps you keep track of your inventory and ensures that you use products within their optimal freshness window.

9. Avoid Contaminants:

- Ensure that containers and tools used for handling extracts are clean and free of contaminants. Contaminants can affect the flavor and safety of the extracts.

10. Regularly Check for Mold or Contamination:

- Periodically inspect your extracts for any signs of mold, discoloration, or contamination. If you notice any issues, discard the affected material to prevent health risks.

11. Use Vacuum-Sealed Packaging:

- Vacuum-sealed packaging can help preserve the freshness of extracts by removing excess air. This is particularly useful for preventing oxidation and maintaining the quality of terpenes.

12. Store in Original Packaging:

- If your extracts come in well-sealed, original packaging, consider keeping them in that packaging to maintain the integrity of the product.

13. Keep Away from Children and Pets:

- Store cannabis extracts in a location that is inaccessible to children and pets. Ensure that the storage area is secure to prevent accidental ingestion.

14. Consult Product-Specific Recommendations:

- Some extracts may come with specific storage recommendations from the manufacturer. Follow these guidelines for optimal storage conditions.

By following these best practices, you can extend the shelf life and preserve the quality of your cannabis extracts, ensuring a more enjoyable and effective experience when you decide to use them.

9.2 Avoiding Degradation

To avoid the degradation of cannabis extracts and preserve their quality over time, consider the following strategies:

1. Temperature Control:

- Store cannabis extracts in a cool environment. High temperatures can accelerate the degradation of cannabinoids and terpenes. Ideally, keep extracts in a dark, cool place, away from direct sunlight and heat sources.

2. Avoid Temperature Fluctuations:

- Minimize temperature fluctuations, as drastic changes can impact the stability of cannabis extracts. Store them in an environment with a consistent temperature to prevent degradation.

3. Dark Storage:

- Exposure to light can degrade cannabinoids and terpenes. Store extracts in opaque containers or dark storage areas to protect them from light-induced degradation.

4. Airtight Containers:

- Use airtight containers to limit exposure to air. Oxygen can oxidize cannabinoids, leading to a loss of potency and changes in flavor. Airtight containers help preserve the quality of the extracts.

5. Avoid Humidity:

- Excessive humidity can contribute to mold growth and degrade the quality of cannabis extracts. Keep the storage environment dry to prevent moisture-related issues.

6. Separate Flavors and Strains:

- If storing multiple extracts, especially with distinct flavors and strains, consider keeping them in separate containers to avoid cross-contamination of aromas and flavors.

7. Refrigeration or Freezing (Depending on Consistency):

- For concentrates like shatter or wax, refrigeration or freezing can help maintain stability. However, avoid freezing extracts with high moisture content, as this can lead to the formation of ice crystals.

8. Labeling:

- Clearly label your extracts with information such as the strain, extraction date, and any other relevant details. This helps you keep track of inventory and ensures that you use products within their optimal freshness window.

9. Avoid Contaminants:

   - Use clean containers and tools for handling extracts to avoid contamination. Contaminants can affect the flavor and safety of the extracts.

10. Regularly Check for Mold or Contamination:

   - Periodically inspect extracts for any signs of mold, discoloration, or contamination. Discard any compromised material to prevent health risks.

11. Use Vacuum-Sealed Packaging:

   - Vacuum-sealed packaging removes excess air, preventing oxidation and preserving the freshness of extracts. This is particularly useful for maintaining the quality of terpenes.

12. Store in Original Packaging:

   - If extracts come in well-sealed, original packaging, consider keeping them in that packaging to maintain the integrity of the product.

13. Avoid Overhandling:

- Minimize unnecessary handling of cannabis extracts to reduce the risk of contamination and exposure to air. Use clean tools and handle extracts with care.

14. Follow Manufacturer Recommendations:

- Some extracts may come with specific storage recommendations from the manufacturer. Follow these guidelines for optimal storage conditions.

By implementing these practices, you can help ensure the longevity and quality of your cannabis extracts, preserving their potency, flavor, and overall effectiveness.

10. LEGALITY AND REGULATIONS

10.1 Global and Regional Perspectives

As of my last knowledge update in January 2022, global and regional perspectives on cannabis vary significantly due to diverse cultural, legal, and societal attitudes. It's important to note that the situation is dynamic, and changes may have occurred since then. Here are general perspectives on cannabis from global and regional standpoints:

Global Perspective:

1. Legalization Trends:

   - The global attitude toward cannabis has been evolving, with an increasing number of countries moving toward some form of cannabis legalization. This includes both medical and recreational use.

2. Medical Cannabis Recognition:

   - Many countries recognize the medicinal properties of cannabis, leading to the establishment of medical cannabis programs. This recognition is driven by scientific research demonstrating the therapeutic potential of cannabinoids.

3. International Cannabis Trade:

- The international cannabis trade has seen growth, with some countries exporting cannabis-related products, including medical cannabis and industrial hemp.

4. Research and Innovation:

- There is a growing interest in cannabis research and innovation globally. Researchers are exploring the potential medical benefits, various strains, and novel delivery methods.

5. Global Cannabis Industry Growth:

- The cannabis industry has experienced significant growth globally, with increased investments, business developments, and the emergence of new products and technologies.

Regional Perspectives:

1. North America:

- The United States and Canada have witnessed substantial developments in cannabis legalization. Several U.S. states have legalized recreational cannabis, while Canada has legalized both medical and recreational use.

2. Europe:

- European countries have diverse attitudes toward cannabis. Some countries, like the Netherlands, have a more lenient approach, while others have strict regulations. Several European countries have established medical cannabis programs.

3. Latin America:

- Some Latin American countries have adopted progressive cannabis policies. Uruguay became the first country to legalize recreational cannabis, and several others have legalized medical use.

4. Asia:

- Many Asian countries maintain strict anti-cannabis policies, and the plant remains illegal in most nations. However, there are discussions and debates about potential policy changes, especially regarding medical cannabis.

5. Africa:

- Cannabis policies in Africa vary widely. Some countries have historically been major producers, while others have strict regulations. There is growing interest in exploring medical cannabis opportunities in certain regions.

6. Oceania:

- Australia and New Zealand have legalized medical cannabis, and there have been discussions about potential changes to recreational cannabis policies. Some Pacific Island nations have a more relaxed attitude toward traditional cannabis use.

7. Middle East:

- The Middle East generally has strict anti-cannabis policies. However, there have been discussions and debates in some countries about potential reforms, especially in the context of medical cannabis.

Considerations:

1. Cultural Factors:

   - Cultural attitudes toward cannabis play a significant role in shaping policies. Some regions have longstanding traditions of cannabis use, while others view it more conservatively.

2. Economic Opportunities:

   - The economic potential of the cannabis industry, including job creation and tax revenues, has influenced policy decisions in various regions.

3. Public Health and Safety:

   - Concerns about public health and safety, including potential impacts on mental health and road safety, often influence the regulatory approach to cannabis.

4. International Agreements:

   - Some countries are bound by international agreements that impact their approach to cannabis. For example, the UN's Single Convention on Narcotic Drugs has influenced drug policies globally.

It's essential to check the latest developments and changes in cannabis policies, as the landscape is evolving. Local laws and attitudes can significantly impact individual experiences with cannabis, whether for medical or recreational purposes.

10.2 Changes in Legislation

As of my last knowledge update in January 2022, the legal status of cannabis was undergoing changes in various regions globally. Please note that developments in cannabis legislation can occur frequently, and there may have been changes since then. It's crucial to verify the latest information from authoritative sources. Here are some general trends and changes observed in cannabis legislation:

Global Trends:

1. Continued Legalization:

   - Several countries and U.S. states have continued to move toward the legalization of cannabis, either for medical or recreational use.

2. Medical Cannabis Expansion:

   - Many regions have expanded access to medical cannabis, recognizing its potential therapeutic benefits. This includes the establishment of medical cannabis programs and the legalization of medical cannabis products.

3. Decriminalization Efforts:

   - Some areas have taken steps to decriminalize the possession of small amounts of cannabis, treating it as a civil offense rather than a criminal one.

4. Industrial Hemp Regulations:

   - Regulations regarding industrial hemp and hemp-derived products, particularly those containing CBD (cannabidiol), have been evolving. Some regions have established clear guidelines for the cultivation and sale of hemp.

Country-Specific Changes:

1. United States:

   - Several U.S. states have legalized recreational cannabis use, and there have been ongoing efforts to pass federal legislation to remove cannabis from the list of controlled substances.

2. Canada:

   - Canada legalized recreational cannabis in 2018, becoming the second country in the world to do so. Since then, the legal cannabis industry has continued to grow.

3. European Union:

   - Some European countries have expanded medical cannabis programs, and there have been discussions at the EU level regarding the standardization of regulations for medical cannabis.

4. South America:

- Some South American countries, including Uruguay and Argentina, have made strides in cannabis legalization for both medical and recreational use.

5. Africa:

- Several African countries have been exploring cannabis legalization and regulatory frameworks. Lesotho, for example, has legalized the cultivation and export of medical cannabis.

6. Asia:

- While many Asian countries maintain strict anti-cannabis policies, there have been discussions and pilot programs exploring medical cannabis in certain regions.

Considerations:

1. Public Opinion:

- Changing public attitudes toward cannabis, influenced by education and awareness, often drive shifts in legislation.

2. Economic Considerations:

- The economic potential of the cannabis industry, including job creation and tax revenues, can influence policy decisions.

3. Medical Research:

- Growing scientific evidence supporting the medical benefits of cannabis has contributed to the expansion of medical cannabis programs.

4. Social Justice:

- Concerns about social justice and the disproportionate impact of cannabis-related arrests on certain communities have prompted calls for cannabis reform.

5. International Agreements:

- Countries may consider their international obligations and agreements when making changes to cannabis legislation.

It's important to check the most recent and specific information regarding cannabis legislation in your jurisdiction. Laws can vary significantly, and developments may have occurred since my last update. Always refer to authoritative sources, government agencies, or legal professionals for the latest information.

11. CANNABIS EXTRACTS AND HEALTH

11.1 Therapeutic Uses

Cannabis and its derivatives have been explored for various therapeutic uses due to the presence of cannabinoids, which interact with the endocannabinoid system in the human body. While research is ongoing, some therapeutic uses of cannabis and its compounds, such as THC (tetrahydrocannabinol) and CBD (cannabidiol), have shown promise. It's important to note that the effectiveness of cannabis for therapeutic purposes can vary, and its use should be approached with caution, particularly under the guidance of healthcare professionals. Here are some therapeutic uses:

1. Pain Management:

- Cannabis, particularly strains with higher levels of THC, has been used for pain relief. It may be beneficial for chronic pain conditions, such as neuropathic pain and arthritis.

2. Anti-Inflammatory Effects:

- Cannabinoids, especially CBD, exhibit anti-inflammatory properties. This makes cannabis a potential option for conditions involving inflammation, such as rheumatoid arthritis.

3. Nausea and Vomiting:

- THC, the psychoactive compound in cannabis, has been used to alleviate nausea and vomiting, particularly in cancer patients undergoing chemotherapy.

4. Appetite Stimulation:

- Cannabis, and specifically THC, is known to stimulate appetite. This can be beneficial for individuals undergoing treatments that suppress appetite, such as cancer patients undergoing chemotherapy.

5. Cancer Symptom Management:

- Cannabis has been explored for managing symptoms related to cancer and its treatments, including pain, nausea, and loss of appetite.

6. Epilepsy and Seizures:

- CBD has shown promise in the treatment of certain forms of epilepsy, leading to the development of the pharmaceutical drug Epidiolex, which is approved for the treatment of specific seizure disorders.

7. Anxiety and Depression:

- Some individuals report that certain strains of cannabis, particularly those with higher CBD content, may help alleviate symptoms of anxiety and depression. However, the relationship between cannabis and mental health is complex, and individual responses can vary.

8. Sleep Disorders:

-   Cannabis, particularly strains with higher levels of THC, may have sedative effects, which could be beneficial for individuals experiencing sleep disorders such as insomnia.

9. Multiple Sclerosis (MS):

-   Cannabis has been explored for managing symptoms of multiple sclerosis, including spasticity and neuropathic pain.

10. Inflammatory Bowel Diseases:

-   Some studies suggest that cannabis may have anti-inflammatory effects that could be beneficial for conditions like Crohn's disease and ulcerative colitis.

11. Glaucoma:

-   Cannabis has been investigated for its potential to reduce intraocular pressure, which is a factor in conditions like glaucoma. However, other more targeted medications are typically preferred for glaucoma treatment.

12. Neuroprotective Properties:

-   Some research suggests that cannabinoids, particularly CBD, may have neuroprotective properties, making them potentially beneficial for conditions involving neurodegeneration.

13. PTSD (Post-Traumatic Stress Disorder):

- Some individuals with PTSD report finding relief from symptoms with the use of cannabis. However, the evidence is still limited, and more research is needed in this area.

14. Addiction Treatment:

- Some studies suggest that cannabis or its components may have potential in the treatment of substance addiction, although more research is needed to understand the mechanisms involved.

11.2 Potential Risks

While cannabis has therapeutic potential, it also poses certain risks, especially when used inappropriately or excessively. It's important for individuals to be aware of these potential risks and exercise caution. Here are some of the potential risks associated with cannabis use:

1. Impaired Cognitive Function:

- Cannabis use, particularly THC, can impair cognitive functions such as memory, attention, and learning. This is of particular concern in individuals, especially adolescents, whose brains are still developing.

2. Mental Health Effects:

- Cannabis use has been associated with an increased risk of mental health issues, including anxiety, depression, and psychosis. It may exacerbate pre-existing mental health conditions.

3. Addiction and Dependence:

- Regular and heavy cannabis use can lead to the development of dependence and addiction. Individuals may experience withdrawal symptoms when trying to reduce or stop cannabis use.

4. Respiratory Issues:

   - Smoking cannabis can have negative effects on the respiratory system, similar to tobacco smoke. Chronic use may lead to bronchitis, coughing, and other respiratory issues.

5. Increased Risk of Accidents:

   - Cannabis use can impair coordination and reaction time, increasing the risk of accidents, particularly when driving or operating heavy machinery.

6. Exacerbation of Psychiatric Disorders:

   - Cannabis use may worsen symptoms in individuals with certain psychiatric disorders, such as schizophrenia or bipolar disorder.

7. Cardiovascular Effects:

   - Cannabis use can lead to an increase in heart rate and blood pressure. This may pose risks, particularly for individuals with cardiovascular issues.

8. Impaired Educational and Occupational Performance:

- Regular cannabis use, especially during adolescence, has been associated with lower educational attainment and impaired occupational functioning.

9. Negative Impact on Motivation:

- Chronic cannabis use may be associated with a decrease in motivation, sometimes referred to as "amotivation."

10. Risk of Lung Cancer:

- While research is ongoing, some studies suggest that long-term, heavy cannabis smoking may be associated with an increased risk of lung cancer.

11. Accidental Ingestion:

- Edible cannabis products, especially those that resemble regular food items, pose a risk of accidental ingestion, particularly in children.

12. Cannabis Hyperemesis Syndrome:

- Some individuals may experience cannabis hyperemesis syndrome, a condition characterized by persistent vomiting and abdominal pain associated with chronic cannabis use.

13. Social and Legal Consequences:

- Cannabis use in certain jurisdictions may have legal consequences. Additionally, it may have social consequences, especially in professional and educational settings.

14. Impact on Pregnancy and Breastfeeding:

- Cannabis use during pregnancy may be associated with adverse effects on fetal development. It is generally advised for pregnant and breastfeeding individuals to avoid cannabis.

15. Interaction with Medications:

- Cannabis can interact with certain medications, either enhancing or diminishing their effects. It's important to consult with healthcare professionals, especially if using cannabis alongside other medications.

12. FAQS FOR BEGINNERS

12.1 Common Questions and Answers

1. Is cannabis legal where I live?

- Cannabis laws vary widely by region. Check the current legal status of cannabis in your specific location. Some places have legalized it for both medical and recreational use, while others may have strict regulations or total prohibition.

2. What is the difference between THC and CBD?

- THC (tetrahydrocannabinol) and CBD (cannabidiol) are two of the main cannabinoids in cannabis. THC is psychoactive and responsible for the "high," while CBD is non-psychoactive and is associated with various therapeutic effects.

3. How does cannabis affect the body?

- Cannabis affects the body through the endocannabinoid system, influencing processes such as mood, appetite, and pain perception. THC and CBD interact with cannabinoid receptors in the brain and body.

4. Can I overdose on cannabis?

- While a cannabis overdose is not fatal, consuming too much can lead to uncomfortable symptoms such as anxiety, paranoia, and nausea. It's essential to consume cannabis responsibly and in moderation.

5. How do I determine the potency of a cannabis product?

- Cannabis potency is often measured in terms of THC and CBD percentages. Check product labels for this information. The method of consumption (smoking, vaping, edibles) can also influence potency and onset of effects.

6. Can I drive after using cannabis?

- Driving under the influence of cannabis is illegal in many places. The psychoactive effects of THC can impair coordination and reaction time. It's recommended to wait until the effects have worn off before driving.

7. Can I use cannabis while pregnant or breastfeeding?

- It is generally advised to avoid cannabis during pregnancy and breastfeeding due to potential risks to fetal and infant development. Consult with healthcare professionals for personalized advice.

8. How can I talk to my doctor about using cannabis for medical purposes?

- Be open and honest with your doctor about your interest in using cannabis for medical reasons. They can provide guidance, discuss potential risks and benefits, and help you make informed decisions.

9. What are the different methods of consuming cannabis?

- Cannabis can be consumed in various ways, including smoking, vaping, edibles, tinctures, topicals, and concentrates. Each method has different onset times and durations of effects.

10. What are terpenes in cannabis?

- Terpenes are aromatic compounds found in cannabis and other plants. They contribute to the plant's scent and may have therapeutic effects. Different strains have distinct terpene profiles.

11. Can cannabis help with anxiety or depression?

- While some individuals report relief from anxiety or depression with cannabis use, it can also exacerbate symptoms in others. The relationship between cannabis and mental health is complex, and its effects vary.

12. How long does cannabis stay in the system?

- The duration cannabis stays in the system depends on factors such as frequency of use, metabolism, and the type of test. THC metabolites can be detected in urine for several weeks.

13. Is CBD legal everywhere?

- CBD legality varies. In many places, CBD derived from hemp (containing less than 0.3% THC) is legal, while CBD from marijuana may be subject to stricter regulations.

14. Can I travel with cannabis?

- Traveling with cannabis is subject to local and international laws. It's essential to research and comply with the regulations of both departure and destination locations.

15. Can I use cannabis with other medications?

- Cannabis can interact with certain medications. Consult with healthcare professionals to assess potential interactions and ensure safe use.

Always stay informed about the latest developments and consult with healthcare professionals or legal authorities for specific guidance related to your circumstances.

13. CONCLUSION

13.1 Recap of Key Points

1. Cannabis Plant:

   - Cannabis is a genus of flowering plants that includes Cannabis sativa, Cannabis indica, and Cannabis ruderalis.

2. Cannabinoids:

   - Cannabinoids are chemical compounds found in cannabis. THC (tetrahydrocannabinol) and CBD (cannabidiol) are the most well-known cannabinoids.

3. Endocannabinoid System:

   - The endocannabinoid system is a biological system in the human body that plays a role in regulating various physiological processes.

4. Definition and Basics:

   - Cannabis extracts are concentrated forms of cannabis that isolate and preserve specific compounds, such as cannabinoids and terpenes.

5. Different Forms:

- Extracts come in various forms, including oils, tinctures, concentrates (shatter, wax), hashish, and more.

6. Extraction Methods:

- Popular extraction methods include solvent-based methods (butane, CO2), solventless methods (rosin pressing), and alcohol extraction.

7. Popular Extracts:

- Hashish, kief, tinctures, and cannabis oil are common extracts with distinct properties and uses.

8. Concentrates:

- Shatter, wax, and other concentrates are highly potent extracts with different consistencies and consumption methods.

Cannabinoids and Terpenes:

9. THC (Tetrahydrocannabinol):

- THC is the psychoactive compound in cannabis, responsible for the "high."

10. CBD (Cannabidiol):

   - CBD is a non-psychoactive cannabinoid with potential therapeutic benefits.

11. Other Cannabinoids:

   - There are many other cannabinoids in cannabis, each with unique effects. Examples include CBG, CBN, and THCV.

12. Terpenes:

   - Terpenes are aromatic compounds that contribute to the flavor and aroma of cannabis. They may also have therapeutic effects.

13. Smoking:

   - Smoking is a traditional method of consuming cannabis. It provides quick onset but may have respiratory risks.

14. Vaporizing:

   - Vaporizing heats cannabis without combustion, reducing the risks associated with smoking.

15. Edibles:

- Edibles are cannabis-infused food products. They have a delayed onset but provide long-lasting effects.

16. Topicals:

- Topical products are applied to the skin and are absorbed locally, providing relief without psychoactive effects.

17. Dabbing:

- Dabbing involves vaporizing cannabis concentrates and is known for its high potency.

Responsible Use and Considerations:

18. Understanding Dosage:

- Start with low doses and gradually increase to understand individual tolerance levels.

19. Risks and Precautions:

- Cannabis use may have potential risks, including impaired cognitive function, mental health effects, and dependence.

20. Responsible Use:

   - Consume cannabis responsibly, be aware of local laws, and consider individual health conditions.

21. Personal Preferences:

   - Cannabis effects vary among individuals. Experiment to find strains and consumption methods that align with personal preferences.

22. Medical Considerations:

   - Consult with healthcare professionals, especially when using cannabis for medical purposes or alongside other medications.

23. Legal Considerations:

   - Be aware of and adhere to local cannabis laws, which can vary widely.

24. Legal Changes:

   - Cannabis laws are evolving globally, with an increasing trend toward legalization for medical and recreational use.

25. Regional Attitudes:

- Attitudes toward cannabis vary regionally, influenced by cultural, economic, and health considerations.

26. Pain Management:

   - Cannabis has potential therapeutic uses, including pain management and anti-inflammatory effects.

27. Anxiety and Depression:

   - Some individuals report relief from anxiety and depression with certain cannabis strains, but effects can vary.

28. Epilepsy and Seizures:

   - CBD has shown promise in the treatment of certain forms of epilepsy.

29. Medical Considerations:

   - Cannabis may be considered for various medical conditions, but individual responses and risks should be assessed by healthcare professionals.

30. Impaired Cognitive Function:

   - Cannabis use can impair memory, attention, and learning.

31. Addiction and Dependence:

   - Regular, heavy cannabis use may lead to dependence and addiction.

32. Respiratory Issues:

   - Smoking cannabis can have negative effects on the respiratory system.

33. Mental Health Effects:

   - Cannabis use may be associated with an increased risk of mental health issues.

34. Social and Legal Consequences:

   - Cannabis use can have legal and social consequences, depending on local laws and regulations.

35. Legal Status:

   - Always be aware of the legal status of cannabis in your specific location.

36. THC vs. CBD:

- Understand the differences between THC and CBD, including their effects and potential therapeutic uses.

37. Cannabis and Driving:

   - Avoid driving under the influence of cannabis, as it can impair coordination and reaction time.

38. Consulting with Healthcare Professionals:

   - If considering cannabis for medical purposes, consult with healthcare professionals for guidance.

39. Terpenes and Cannabinoids:

   - Familiarize yourself with terpenes and cannabinoids to understand the effects of different cannabis strains.

40. Responsible Consumption:

   - Consume cannabis responsibly, taking into account individual tolerance levels and potential risks.

Remember that information on cannabis is subject to change, and it's crucial to stay informed about the latest developments and research findings. If in doubt, consult with healthcare professionals or legal authorities for personalized advice.

13.2 Encouragement for Responsible Consumption

Encouraging responsible consumption of cannabis is essential for individuals seeking to incorporate it into their lifestyles. Here are some words of encouragement:

1. Knowledge is Empowerment:

   - Educate yourself about cannabis, including its effects, potential risks, and legal considerations. Being well-informed empowers you to make responsible decisions.

2. Start Low, Go Slow:

   - If you're new to cannabis or trying a new product, start with a low dose and gradually increase. This helps you gauge your tolerance and minimize the risk of overconsumption.

3. Know Your Limits:

   - Understand your personal limits and how cannabis affects you. Pay attention to how different strains, consumption methods, and doses impact your experience.

4. Choose the Right Setting:

   - Consume cannabis in a comfortable and safe environment. Consider your surroundings and who you're with to ensure a positive experience.

5. Consider Your Health:

   - If you have underlying health conditions or are taking medications, consult with healthcare professionals before using cannabis. Consider potential interactions and how it may impact your health.

6. Avoid Driving Under the Influence:

   - Cannabis can impair coordination and reaction time. Never drive or operate heavy machinery under the influence. Use alternative transportation methods when needed.

7. Respect Legal Boundaries:

   - Be aware of and respect local cannabis laws. Responsible use includes adhering to legal regulations to avoid legal consequences.

8. Be Mindful of Others:

   - Be considerate of those around you, especially in shared spaces. Not everyone may be comfortable with cannabis use, so respect others' boundaries and preferences.

9. Take Breaks as Needed:

- Regularly evaluate your cannabis use and consider taking breaks if needed. This can help prevent tolerance build-up and dependency.

10. Stay Hydrated and Nourished:

- Cannabis may affect appetite and hydration. Remember to stay hydrated and maintain a balanced diet to support your overall well-being.

11. Seek Professional Guidance:

- If you're using cannabis for medical purposes or have specific health concerns, consult with healthcare professionals. They can provide personalized guidance based on your individual needs.

12. Mindful Consumption:

- Practice mindfulness when consuming cannabis. Be present in the moment and pay attention to how it affects your mind and body.

13. Cultivate Positive Experiences:

- Use cannabis in a way that enhances your life and well-being. Whether for relaxation, creativity, or medical purposes, focus on cultivating positive experiences.

14. Encourage Open Communication:

- Foster open communication with friends, family, or peers about your cannabis use. Discussing your experiences and concerns can help create a supportive environment.

15. Know When to Seek Help:

- If you ever feel overwhelmed or experience negative effects, don't hesitate to seek help or talk to someone you trust. Responsible consumption includes recognizing when you may need support.

Remember that responsible cannabis use is about making informed choices that align with your health, lifestyle, and legal obligations. By approaching cannabis use with mindfulness and consideration, you can create positive and enjoyable experiences.

Glossary

Key terms and definitions.

Certainly! Here are key terms and definitions related to cannabis and cannabis extracts:

1. Cannabis:

   - A genus of flowering plants that includes Cannabis sativa, Cannabis indica, and Cannabis ruderalis. Cannabis is known for its psychoactive and medicinal properties.

2. Cannabinoids:

   - Chemical compounds found in cannabis. The two main cannabinoids are THC (tetrahydrocannabinol) and CBD (cannabidiol), each with distinct effects.

3. Endocannabinoid System (ECS):

   - A biological system in the human body that plays a role in regulating various physiological processes, including mood, appetite, and pain perception.

4. Cannabis Extracts:

   - Concentrated forms of cannabis that isolate and preserve specific compounds, such as cannabinoids and terpenes.

5. THC (Tetrahydrocannabinol):

   - The psychoactive compound in cannabis responsible for the "high" or euphoric effects.

6. CBD (Cannabidiol):

   - A non-psychoactive cannabinoid with potential therapeutic benefits, such as anti-inflammatory and anti-anxiety effects.

7. Terpenes:

   - Aromatic compounds found in cannabis and other plants that contribute to the plant's scent and may have therapeutic effects.

8. Endocannabinoid Receptors:

   - Receptors in the endocannabinoid system that interact with cannabinoids. CB1 receptors are primarily found in the brain, while CB2 receptors are more prevalent in the immune system.

9. Entourage Effect:

- The theory that cannabinoids and terpenes work synergistically, enhancing each other's therapeutic effects when consumed together.

10. Cannabis Strain:

- A specific variety or type of cannabis plant with unique characteristics, including cannabinoid and terpene profiles.

11. Solvent-Based Extraction:

- A method of extracting cannabinoids and terpenes from cannabis using solvents such as butane, CO_2, or ethanol.

12. Solventless Extraction:

- Extraction methods that do not use external solvents. Rosin pressing is an example of a solventless extraction method.

13. Hashish:

- A concentrated form of cannabis made by compressing and heating trichomes, resulting in a resinous substance.

14. Kief:

- The resinous trichomes that are separated from the cannabis plant and often collected in a fine powder form.

15. Tinctures:

- Liquid extracts of cannabis, typically alcohol-based, that can be consumed sublingually.

16. Concentrates:

- Highly potent cannabis extracts, including forms like shatter, wax, budder, and live resin.

17. Shatter:

- A translucent, glass-like cannabis concentrate with high levels of THC.

18. Wax:

- A cannabis concentrate with a soft, waxy consistency, often high in THC.

19. Dabbing:

- The process of vaporizing and inhaling concentrated cannabis extracts using a hot surface.

20. Edibles:

   - Cannabis-infused food products that deliver cannabinoids when consumed.

21. Vaporizing (Vaping):

   - The inhalation of vaporized cannabis using a device that heats the material without combustion.

22. Topicals:

   - Cannabis-infused products such as creams, balms, or lotions applied to the skin for localized relief without psychoactive effects.

23. Cannabis Oil:

   - An extract of cannabis that is typically consumed orally, either directly or added to food or beverages.

24. Cannabinoid Receptor Agonist:

   - Substances that activate cannabinoid receptors in the endocannabinoid system, mimicking the effects of cannabinoids.

25. Cannabinoid Receptor Antagonist:

- Substances that block or inhibit the activation of cannabinoid receptors in the endocannabinoid system.

26. Microdosing:

- Consuming very low doses of cannabis to achieve subtle therapeutic effects without the typical psychoactive experience.

27. Cannabis Hyperemesis Syndrome:

- A condition characterized by persistent vomiting and abdominal pain associated with chronic cannabis use.

28. Medical Cannabis:

- Cannabis used for medical purposes, often prescribed by healthcare professionals to manage specific health conditions.

29. Recreational Cannabis:

- Cannabis used for non-medical purposes, often for enjoyment or relaxation.

30. Legalization:

- The process of making cannabis use, cultivation, or distribution permissible by law.

31. Decriminalization:

   - The reduction or removal of legal penalties for cannabis possession or use without fully legalizing it.

32. Dispensary:

   - A legal retail establishment where cannabis products are sold, often for medical or recreational use.

33. Terpene Profile:

   - The combination and concentration of different terpenes in a particular cannabis strain, contributing to its unique aroma and potential effects.

These terms provide a foundation for understanding the various aspects of cannabis, its extracts, and the broader cannabis culture. Always stay informed about developments in cannabis research and regulations, as the field is dynamic and evolving.